Praise for
Ayahuasca: An Executive's Enlightenment

"This book is more than Ayahuasca. It's an existential peek into the question we all ask ourselves: Why am I here? What is my purpose? Michael explores this incredible thirst for enlightenment and helps us unleash the unlimited potential inside all of us."

—Mark W. Guay, host of *Your Life On Purpose*

"Ayahuasca: An Executive's Enlightenment is the most authentic story of a person uncovering themselves that I've ever read. I found it inspirational, hopeful and honest. An important reminder that the paths to self-discovery aren't always the traditional ones."

—Duncan Penn, *The Buried Life* and Co-Author of Best-Selling *What Do You Want to Do Before You Die?*

"There are people who have experienced profound spiritual epiphanies and have the extraordinary gift to convey the power and wisdom found in transcendent states. Sanders has that gift. We travel with him into the world of Ayahuasca and the mystical journey that changes his life, forever. *Ayahuasca: An Executive's Enlightenment* is infused with the spirit of Ayahuasca and will work its magic on you, as it has on me. "

—Dr. Sherrill Sellman, N.D. & Best-Selling Author of *Hormone Heresy: What Women MUST Know About their Hormones*

"Ayahuasca: An Executive's Enlightenment smacks of authenticity. Sanders places you in the jungle with its smells, sounds, tastes and sights, and weaves a splendid story about his Ayahuasca experience."

—Stanley Krippner, Professor of Psychology at Saybrook University and Co-Author of *Demystifying Shamans and their World*

"Sanders' sincerity is palpable from cover to cover, and I recommend the read to anyone interested in getting to know Mother Ayahuasca, or for anyone seeking inspiration and understanding in general. *Ayahuasca: An Executive's Enlightenment* not only brought back important insights and memories, but also exposed me to ideas I had never considered before."

—Jason Abbott, host of *Intellectual Gentlemen's Club*

AYAHUASCA

AN EXECUTIVE'S ENLIGHTENMENT

MICHAEL SANDERS

Printed in the United States of America

First Printing, 2015

978-0-9948264-0-4 (paperback)
978-0-9948264-1-1 (ebook)

Sage & Feather Press
Toronto, Canada

AYAHUASCA

AN EXECUTIVE'S ENLIGHTENMENT

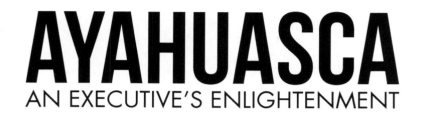

MICHAEL SANDERS

This book is dedicated to the infinite
potential inside all of us.

ACKNOWLEDGMENTS

Thank you to:
Guy Crittenden for his editing, feedback, and guidance throughout the writing process.

Mark Nabeta, Rob Sanders, Stephanie Ligeti, Chris Toman, Sky Curtis, and Dan Cleland for editing and providing valuable feedback.

Maria D'Marco for helping me tell my story.

Stanley Krippner for his insights and support.

Matt Gray, Scott Oldford, and Tyler Benjamin Wagner for their sage advice in how to go about publishing and connecting with wider audiences.

Guy Vincent for providing the Publishizer platform to make this book a reality.

Vinsu Tran and Kit Knows for their video production and creative expertise.

Peter Barlow for his design work.

Dan, Tatyana, and Victor for operating such an incredible trip. Also, Dan and Tatyana for filming interviews with the members of our group, which helped in my recollection of the others' ceremonial experiences.

Jon, Carl, and Sid for being part of the experience and wonderful friends.

Ricardo, Erjomenes, Ersilia, Rafa, and Ana for guiding me during this spiritual journey.

Mother Ayahuasca.

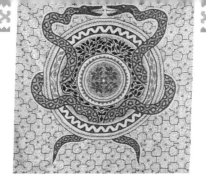

A Loving Thanks and Infinite Gratitude for the following Patrons who made Special Contributions to the Crowdfunding Campaign for *Ayahuasca: An Executive's Enlightenment*:

Guy Vincent
Franz Schwennicke
Alexandra Hastings
Wil Eitel
Iain Davis
Michael Weissman
Pam & Dave Sanders
Rob Sanders
Neal De Florio
Sidney Smith
Stephane Ouellette
Harrison Singer
Calan Aldred
Alyssa Alikpala
Stacey Alvarez
Ayelet Baron
Giovanni Bartolomeo
Russell Boyd
Kelly Breckon
Rob Creighton
Guy Crittenden
Nick Demco
Logan Desrosiers
Tom Dudderidge
Edward Frezza

Mike Hall
Brittany Kaminski
Stephanie Ligeti
Ian McArthur
Harrison Milborne
Daniel Millard
Jo Morin
Drummond Munro
Victor Neumann
David Niry
Scott Oldford
Lara Pedrini
Scott Purkis
Ron Scarafile
Graham Scott
Ian Scott
Lili Sie
Christopher Sinnott
Timothy Sotoadeh
Mark Szilard
Tatyana Telegina
Jasmine Vegso
Domenic Venneri
Mike Wainstock

A NOTE TO THE READER

Throughout my time in Peru, I experienced things I would have previously thought unreal.

With this book, I am sharing with you an incredible and transformative experience, one that I hope inspires you to become the person you've always wanted to be—the person you've always known you truly are.

With love,
Michael Sanders

FEBRUARY 2, 2013

My strength is low, my vigor gone, and my libido shot. I sleep at least ten hours each night and never feel rested. I'm working as the vice president of an advertising agency and the co-founder of a separate start-up in the gaming industry, but I'm just going through the motions. The only things I look forward to are my next workout and falling asleep. I'm training athletically ten to fourteen times each week—something I once found joy in, but now borders on addiction. I enjoy seeing friends, but it takes enormous effort. My zest for living is on the verge of disappearing, and if I can't start feeling like myself again within two years, I'm going to put a bullet in my brain.

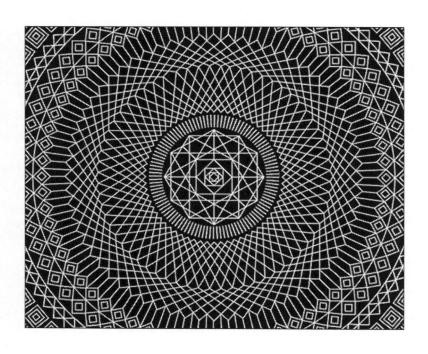

DECEMBER 27, 2013

I arrive at the Golden Star Hotel in downtown Iquitos, Peru with two of my best friends, Sid and Carl. The three of us met seven years ago during our first week at The University of Western Ontario. While we were close right from the get-go, our bond deepened when my best friend, Dave, fell to his death from a fifteen-story balcony in a tragic accident on October 17, 2010. Shortly thereafter, Carl, Sid and I each relocated to Toronto, the city we now call home.

Carl is muscular like a bull and an incredible athlete. He captained the university rugby team and, during his teens, competed at a national level in badminton. He's now a sales executive and has perhaps the most systematic mind I've encountered. Each decision he makes is a calculated one, and each situation an opportunity for him to achieve a goal. Carl has an astounding voice and one of his current goals is to share his music with the world.

Sid, on the other hand, is much more free-flowing. A savvy entrepreneur who runs a division of his family's wholesale and distribution company, Sid globetrots in search of both business opportunities and personal pleasure. Shaggy-haired and of average build, Sid is also known as Sods, a nickname our friends use to describe him when he enters party mode. To Sods, it's like the rest of the world doesn't exist. He completely shuts it out and lives only in the present moment. Sid also has an uncanny ability to quickly form deep and lasting friendships with the most wonderful people.

Inside the hotel, we are given a warm welcome from Sid's childhood friend and tour leader, Dan Cleland. Dan, a tall and handsome young man from Canada, runs a company called Pulse Tours that offers various excursions throughout South America, some of which revolve around the Amazonian tradition of Ayahuasca.

After getting settled into our room, we head down to the restaurant for an orientation meeting.

We meet Dan's girlfriend, Tatyana, a blonde, blue-eyed, beautiful 21-year-old Canadian citizen originally from Kazakhstan and Victor, a five-foot, six-inch man with dark skin, an athletic build, and a small pot belly. Victor hails from Iquitos and will act as our jungle guide.

We meet two other men, Jon and Guy, who, like us, have travelled to Peru to embark on this adventure with Pulse Tours. Dark-skinned and slender, Jon is a 26-year-old Filipino with a shaved head, who now lives in Florida. Guy, 53, lives not far from Toronto. He's tall, with an average build for his age, and has a bald head, goatee, an earring in his left ear, and wears glasses. Guy co-founded and edits two environmental magazines and is the father of two boys.

Dan explains the trip's itinerary, which includes trekking through the jungle, boating down the Amazon River, and to my surprise, three Ayahuasca ceremonies. I expected to take part in only two ceremonies—thinking that would be more than enough—but after speaking with the group, I become comfortable with the idea of three.

Ayahuasca, often referred to as "Mother Ayahuasca", is a psychedelic and medicinal beverage brewed from the

Banisteriopsis caapi vine and, in our case, chacruna leaves containing dimethyltryptamine (DMT). I first heard of the plant medicine in early 2012 while listening to an episode of The Joe Rogan Experience podcast. During the episode, Joe chatted with Aubrey Marcus about Aubrey's recent trip to the Amazon where he met Mother Ayahuasca. The details of Aubrey's experience were profound. He spoke of overcoming past traumas and fears by vomiting suppressed memories into a bucket. He recounted having an out-of-body experience, during which he removed a gooey liquid from the glands in his neck to alleviate a chronic swelling he had suffered his entire life. He mentioned accessing other dimensions as well. Though the story seemed unbelievable, the tone in Aubrey's voice and the way he articulated the events, suggested he was telling the truth.

Having always been fascinated with the exploration of consciousness, I knew then that I would, at some point, encounter the strange psychedelic brew. It wasn't until my return from Burning Man[1] in September 2013 that I learned how this would happen.

* * *

"Mike, what are you doing for New Year's?" Sid asks me.

"Nothing planned yet, brother," I tell him.

"Ok, well, I want to do something different. I don't want to go to a house party and drink. I want to explore."

---

1   Burning Man is an annual weeklong festival held around Labor Day in the Black Rock desert of Nevada. The Burning Man organization creates the infrastructure of Black Rock City, wherein 70,000 participants (a.k.a. "Burners") dedicate themselves to the spirit of community, art, self-expression, and self-reliance. They depart one week later, leaving no trace. As simple as this may seem, trying to explain what Burning Man is to someone who has never been to the event is like trying to explain a kaleidoscope to a blind person. To truly understand this event, one must participate. (Burningman.com)

"What do you have in mind?"

"My friend Dan has been living in and taking people on expeditions throughout South America for the past few years and I've been meaning to get down there. Recently, he's been taking people to discover this plant medicine called Ayahuasca. Have you heard of it?" Sid asks.

"Oh man, yes! Yes! I've been listening to podcasts about it. I'm in, man. I'm in! It sounds like the craziest trip ever!"

"I know, right!? But, I don't think it's really a recreational experience," Sid explains. "It involves ceremony and shamans, and they treat it as a medicine, not a drug. Apparently, a specific diet needs to be followed leading up to drinking the Ayahuasca, and with each ceremony you're encouraged to set an intention— something that you want to work on. The Ayahuasca helps you figure out your intention, whether it relates to your career, relationships, or something else. I read that the medicine will show you what you need to be shown, even if you don't know what it is that you're looking for."

"You've been doing your research, I see. I'll start researching more deeply myself, but either way, I'm in."

* * *

Amazonian Peruvians have been using the Ayahuasca brew for millennia for divinatory and healing purposes, treating a diverse range of conditions from depression to cancer. With the brew's ability to provide its drinkers with clarity about life and our universe, many Westerners have referred to it as "thirty years worth of psychotherapy in a cup."

A specific *dieta*[2] avoiding salt, spices, red meat, pork, alcohol, drugs, sex and orgasm should be practiced for a week or two leading up to ceremony, and those apprenticing with shamans will practice the dieta for much longer durations. Ayahuasca is said to have a female spirit, and while I'm skeptical of a plant having a female spirit, and of the need to modify my diet, I remain open-minded enough to respect the folklore and practice the customs.

After the meeting, Dan, Tatyana, Jon, Guy, Carl, Sid, and I board a boat to eat lunch at *Del Fria al Fuego* (a.k.a. Floating Restaurant), a two-story restaurant with a swimming pool that floats in the middle of the river.

On the ride over, Jon asks me about my intention with Ayahuasca.

"Hmm. I haven't really solidified an intention," I say, "but I'd like to find some clarity on my career path. I'm also interested to learn more about my body, so that I can re-train certain neuromuscular pathways to prevent the symptoms of past injuries from resurfacing. How about you? What's your intention?"

"I'm here for a karmic cleanse. I've been clearing my karma lately, and I just want to keep clearing."

"Cool," I say, not entirely sure what he's talking about.

"When's your birthday?" Jon asks.

"St. Patrick's Day, March 17th," I reply.

---

2   "Dieta", which translates as "diet", means that a shaman or shaman-in-training consumes a particular plant, usually on a daily basis and accompanied by a specific nutritional protocol, as a way of connecting with the plant and learning from its teachings. According to Peruvian shamans, plants have a double function. They may be used as medicinal plants for various illnesses or they can function as plant teachers, if used under the special conditions of diet and segregation (http://www.elmundomagico.org/shamanic-plant-diet/).

Jon's eyes light up.

"See this tattoo?" He turns to show me the back of his neck, which reads *Sleepy Bear*. "That's for my ex-boyfriend. He died about a year ago. His birthday was March 17th."

"Ah man, I'm sorry. Did you get that tattoo after he died?"

"No, I got it when we were still together—a few years ago."

"Whoa. So, you got the *Sleepy Bear* tattoo before he went for the ultimate sleep? Did he sleep a lot?"

"Yeah, he slept a lot," Jon says.

"Seems prophetic."

"Yeah." Jon smiles.

At the restaurant, I eat fresh ceviche and smoke a few mapachos, the sacred South American tobacco. The buzz is electric, and being a rare tobacco smoker, the mapacho shoots me close to the moon; a little more potent than a nice Cuban cigar.

Dan sits across from me and I ask how he likes running Pulse Tours.

"Man, overall, it's amazing. Some days, I know there's nothing I'd rather do. When somebody has a life-changing experience, it's rewarding. A guy on a recent trip—his name's Geoffrey, and you'll meet him once we get to the ceremonial place—told me that I helped him discover a part of himself he thought he had lost a long time ago. So, I mean, that..." Dan's eyes light up. "That was awesome. But, other days are a struggle. On our last trip, a woman left early because she was so unhappy. She thought I had planned too much into the trip. She was upset about the road conditions, she had a bad Ayahuasca experience, and she blamed me for it. She left after the first ceremony, and I paid to re-arrange her travel plans. I actually lost money on her."

"She blamed her bad Ayahuasca experience on you? Perhaps she just didn't have the right mindset," I suggest. "Sounds to me like you should focus your energy on the people like Geoffrey and not worry about the odd person who's upset by a muddy road. It's a jungle experience, after all! I'm only a few hours in, but I feel like you've got something special here."

"I appreciate that."

Back in the city, we shop for local goods and gifts. The street jewelers persuade us to peruse their work, much of it beautiful. We wander into large stores with many vendors. Some from our group buy jewelry; others purchase clothing for the ceremonies. I buy a pair of comfortable and loose-fitting blue pants while keeping an eye out for gifts for Linnea, my lovely girlfriend. Thinking this will be my last opportunity to purchase anything prior to disappearing into the jungle, I'm keen to find something nice for my love. Tatyana helps me choose a beautiful blue-feathered earring; and after a lot of browsing, one of the vendors shows me a bracelet that I know will be perfect. I negotiate with the storeowner and make my purchases.

After shopping, our group sits down for dinner at a restaurant called *Dawn on the Amazon*, owned by Bill Grimes, a graying man from Indiana, who came to Iquitos twenty years ago in search of adventure. The food is delicious and some of the guys enjoy beer and mapachos.

At the other end of the table, Jon and Tatyana speak about precious rocks.

"Something's different about your energy," Tatyana says to Jon.

"You noticed? I've felt different ever since I put on this necklace," Jon replies, referring to the necklace he bought earlier.

I think about rolling my eyes, but choose to refrain from judgment. Their conversation shifts to numerology.

"That's where I draw the line," Carl mutters to me and smirks. "Ooh... there are eights everywhere. So what? There are other numbers too. Fuckin' numerology. Pfft."

I'm inclined to agree, but hold off on a conclusion.

Guy, Tatyana, and Jon then start talking about Reiki, and I chuckle to myself, thinking about how alienating this New Age talk might be for some of my friends back home.

DECEMBER 28, 2013

Satiated from the pistachios I ate before bed, I skip breakfast and practice handstands and gymnastics instead. Once the others finish their morning meal, Victor escorts us to the Belen Market, the largest traditional market in the Peruvian Amazon.

A concoction of hundreds of odors assaults my nostrils: raw meat of all kinds, tobacco, fish, vegetables, blood, spices, people, sweat, plastic, steel, rainwater, garbage, dogs, cotton, babies, flowers, farts, alcohol, and rubber. Families, each with a particular niche—whether selling tortoise meat, beef, cigarettes or flip-flops—have tables set up to showcase their goods. Butchers hack at animals, both dead and alive; getting squirted with rodent blood is not unexpected.

Peruvians saunter through the crowded aisles; we are the only gringos in sight. Victor hands each of us a natural mint, a tiny white egg-shaped object with a hard core that's meant to be sucked on. I fumble mine, dropping it to the wet and muddy ground. Victor is quick to hand me another, and it tastes all right. A dark-skinned Peruvian man picks up a raw chicken and inspects it before tossing the dead bird back into the pile.

"This place disgusts me," says Carl with a scowl, and Sid and I laugh. My leg rubs against a giant wet fish that's hanging off the edge of a woman's table as drops of rainwater slide through the canopies above onto my shoulder. It's a bright sunny morning following a rainy night.

People aren't particularly fit in Iquitos, but their faces are warm with happiness. I smile at a little girl holding her mom's hand as they stroll around gathering their day's groceries. Many city blocks in size, the Belen Market dwarfs any Costco.

Victor takes us through a building, what I presume to be someone's home, to a boat just outside the market. We climb aboard the long and narrow vessel, much like a large canoe, with a small motor at the back and a canopy made of straw-like material to shield passengers from the sun and rain.

We then boat through the city.

In Iquitos, the water levels fluctuate up to fifteen meters through the different seasons, so in many areas people build their homes on stilts. In July, the locals might walk to their neighbors, but come February, they either have to swim or boat. We see people hanging laundry, eating food, and bathing in the river as we motor by.

We cruise out of the city and hop into a van that already has our luggage strapped to its top. We drive for about an hour under beautiful blue and sunny skies, wispy clouds floating over the green jungle trees, before we stop at the Peruvian equivalent of a highway service center. Two women and a young girl manage a charcoal-powered grill. We place our orders and sit at picnic tables inside a wooden structure that backs onto a jungle expanse. While we wait for our food, children dance and play in the back. A whole fish and half a chicken are delivered to me. Each bite makes me salivate, and I wish that Canadian service centers served such caliber of food. Tatyana spots a stand with young coconuts and orders, "Un coco, por favor."

"Dos cocos," Dan chimes in.

"Tres cocos," Jon says.

"Cuatro cocos," Guy pipes up.

"Cinco cocos," I say. Carl asks if I can get him one, and I know Sid will want one too.

"Umm, dos more cocos, por favor," I ask, as I hold up two fingers to the woman, unsure how "six" and "seven" translate to Spanish. The lady smiles, hands me three coconuts, and I take a sip from one of them.

We drive a bit longer before the eight of us climb aboard another riverboat, en route to our jungle lodge via the Amazon River.

Jon asks me questions about fitness and movement. He's inexperienced with athletic physicality, but is keen on better connecting with his body. We chat about mobility, weightlifting, gymnastics, basketball, snowboarding, rock climbing, yoga, and dance before the conversation transitions to nutrition.

"So, you eat a lot of meat?" he asks.

"Yeah, you could say that."

"Why?"

"Health and performance reasons."

"See, I just started as a raw vegan, but I don't know what it's like to be an athlete. You think you need to eat the meat?" he asks.

"Well, yeah, there are essential B vitamins and amino acids that humans can only get from meat."

"Hmm, I don't know about that," Jon says, sounding almost skeptical.

"Well, there might be ways to skirt around that with precise supplementation, but I prefer to focus on eating real food. I know some serious athletes who have tried raw veganism for a year or two. Initially, it worked quite well for them, but over time, they became injured and depressed."

"Why do you think that is?"

"They just weren't getting what their bodies needed."

"So, do you at least eat organic?" Jon asks.

"Yeah. I go straight to the farmers who raise their cows, bison, elk, and lamb on grass with humane practices. The animals lead healthy lives."

"So, the only darkness they endure is the death itself…"

"Yes. But, I don't necessarily see death as darkness. I don't perceive life and death as a dichotomy, but rather a transition from one stage to the next; and I'm respectful of the animal that nourishes me and allows me to be my best."

"Interesting. For me, I just don't want that karma. And, when I switched to raw vegan, I felt so much better."

"Well, what was your diet like before?"

"Pretty awful." He laughs.

"That's the thing. Anybody who switches from a Standard American Diet (SAD) to a more health-conscious diet will experience heightened clarity and better health. You're eliminating so many toxins from your diet."

"Ah, good point," Jon says. "Again, I don't know what it's like to be an athlete, but there's a guy who lives just off breathing, and another who lives just off light. All of it has to do with belief."

Now, *I'm* becoming skeptical. "Hmm, I'd have to see that to believe it. Ultimately though, if raw veganism makes you feel good, then stick with it. Everybody's different."

We arrive at the confluence of the Ucayali and the Maranon Rivers, where the Amazon officially begins[3], and Sid asks Victor if it's safe to swim.

"Yes, of course," says Victor in his rhythmic Peruvian accent, as he looks up from his *Birds of the Amazon* book. The group doesn't seem convinced. Half-joking inquiries about piranhas and alligators are made, but Victor assures us we'll be safe. "You're

---

3   The Amazon actually begins as a trickle from a glacier near Arequipa, but the officially named Amazon River begins at this place where the Ucayali and Maranon merge.

fine as long as you swim mid-river. The animals that might bother you live closer to the banks."

I strip off my tank top and dive into the brown Amazon water. Dan follows suit, and then Carl, Sid, and Guy jump in as well.

"We didn't come all this way to *not* swim in the Amazon!" I shout. I front crawl, tread, breaststroke, backstroke, somersault, and butterfly through the river as a trio of currents converging near our boat pulls me in a few other directions. My skin feels crisp, my body nimble, and my soul alive! The five of us in the water laugh and splash around, and I think we all appreciate our capacity to deal with the currents. *Swimming in the Amazon: wow!* One by one, we climb back aboard the boat before continuing on our journey.

With four hours of traveling under our belts, we bank the boat and arrive to our home for the next few days: a rustic jungle lodge consisting of eight or nine small wooden structures linked together by wooden bridges. Everything is elevated on stilts.

Carl, Sid, and I take our room: a pale-green square space about four hundred square feet, with three beds protected by mosquito nets, a table to place belongings, screens for windows, and a clothes line running through the middle. A toilet, shower and sink are at the back. I wouldn't have been disappointed to see a squatting toilet, but this jungle lodge has near first-world plumbing and fixtures. We each claim a bed before Carl and I take a stroll of the land.

We walk along a perfectly level concrete sidewalk that surrounds the village and soccer field that neighbor our lodge. The inhabitants of each and every home smile and wave as we pass by. We veer off the path through some tall plants, run into a rooster who scurries in fear, and then find the river's edge. A pair of young boys, probably six and eight, have their rods cast in the water waiting for a bite. Carl bends over and picks up what appears to be a handcrafted walking stick and we head back to the sidewalk. A giant vulture tree grows from the river's bank and eight of the black birds perch on its branches. On the other side of the river, about fifteen white birds sit on the bank and another fifteen fly above it.

"I feel vultures," Carl says.

"I figured you would, Mamma.[4] They're pretty cool. I prefer the white birds though," I respond.

"Yeah, doesn't surprise me."

"Dude, do you think Peruvians are happier than North Americans?"

"They don't have much, but they seem pretty smiley," Carl says.

"Agreed. It's hard to tell as a tourist passing through though. I mean, very few people—in Canada or Peru—walk around broadcasting unhappiness. People rarely talk about their shortcomings or insecurities the first time you meet them, so sometimes I wonder if we're just seeing a surface happiness. But then, I get this deeper sense that these people, in general, are genuinely happier than North Americans."

An old man with his hands clasped behind his back walks past us, smiles, and says "Ola," and we return the gesture.

Back at the lodge, I find Sid with his shaggy hair and beard in one of the gazebo's hammocks. I lie down on another hammock and he and I watch the sun descend in the sky as it paints pink and orange beams across a blue and white canvas.

When it's nearly dark outside, Victor pops his head in and says, "Dinner is ready." His sensual accent sounds like music to our ears. Chicken, vegetables, and rice are served in the dining room as our group of eight assembles for a family-style meal. Dan, Guy, and Victor each have a beer.

---

4   "Mamma" is a nickname my group of friends calls Carl—not to be confused with "Mamma Ayahuasca".

"You're not worried about the alcohol interfering with your Ayahuasca experience?" Sid asks.

"Nah man, we've got three days before the ceremonies," Dan says, as Tatyana rolls her eyes.

"I'm just following Dan's lead." Guy says with a big grin, barely able to contain his laughter.

Dan then shares that he's participated in eighteen Ayahuasca ceremonies. When we inquire about the details, he recounts bright colors, geometric patterns, the vomiting and other purging, and the loving visions he's had of family members while under Mother Ayahuasca's care.

"I learned that I need to be a more supportive brother and son, and it has really improved my relationships with family members, so I'm very grateful for that," Dan says. "I actually brought my dad down here earlier this year. It was too bad, though: we drank this vomit-inducing remedy before our scheduled Ayahuasca ceremony—something the shamans[5] recommend as a cleansing tool prior to taking the Ayahuasca itself. It ended up making my dad feel sick, and he didn't feel well enough to drink Ayahuasca. That was pretty disappointing, but it was great to have him down here, no less."

Following dinner, we prepare for a nighttime jungle trek by getting into pants, long sleeves, and rubber boots. The others apply mosquito repellant, but I refrain. For the past few years, mosquitoes and their bites haven't bothered me, and the repellant seems to work more like an attractant. This shift occurred four years ago when I switched my diet to one consisting only of vegetables, meat, seafood, fruit, nuts, eggs, and rice.

---

5   In Peru, the Ayahuasca healers typically refer to themselves as curanderos or ayahuasqueros; however, as knowledge of the brew spreads globally, shaman has become more or less interchangeable with the other two terms.

While filling my water bottle, my stomach rumbles and I run to the washroom to diarrhea. I'm forced to make three trips in the span of twenty-five minutes, and I hope this disturbance doesn't persist throughout the night.

I emerge from our room to see Sid playing with a giant, hairy, pink-footed tarantula. Carl handles it too. After a slight apprehension, I let the furry creature crawl around my arms and hands for a few seconds before passing it off.

We hop aboard our boat and venture out onto the Amazon underneath a starry night sky and I'm exposed to constellations I haven't seen before. So far from any city's light pollution, the distant balls of fire shine bright into my eyes and I recognize layers upon layers of celestial bodies. Every time I gaze at stars above, I feel small, big, infinite and connected all at the same time, and tonight on the Ucayali is no different.

We pull our boat up onto the bank and disembark. My stomach churns and I hope that I don't shit my pants. Victor and his small, agile friend, Alipio, lead us through head-high plants and into an open expanse in the middle of the jungle. Gigantic trees surround us and the sounds of crickets and thousands of other insects play in tandem for our ears. We shine our flashlights in hopes of seeing animals as Victor waves us over to check out another hairy tarantula ascending a tree.

"Sanders, should we turn this into a real adventure?" Carl looks at me.

"You want to leave the group and explore the jungle on our own, Mamma?" I ask.

"Yeah man, we don't need these guides. Fuck it."

"Maybe we'll befriend a jaguar or something."

Carl and I walk between some trees and push past the leaves of giant plants in a direction different from our group's. Twenty meters into our mission, we pause at the edge of an area of dense brush. I look at Carl and our grins reveal that we weren't committed to this independent excursion. When we catch up to the group, Carl says, "We were going to ditch you guys, but Sanders pussied out."

On the lookout for more creatures, Victor spots a black scorpion and warns us to take care in our approach. He then disables the scorpion with the side of his machete and carefully picks it up by the tail to avoid getting stung. Lifting the animal up, he explains, "This scorpion can kill you."

My stomach continues to growl. I resolve not to drink any more water and turn my thoughts to Linnea to take my mind away from the upset brewing in my intestines.

Victor shows us some tree frogs, more spiders, and various insects. Despite the fact that there are nine flashlights, only Victor's and Alipio's ever discover creatures.

"Do not touch anything around here," Victor cautions, standing beside a tree that crawls with red ants. "These are the fire ants, and if they bite you, it burns. It burns so bad. In Peru, if a man cheats on his wife or girlfriend, the people take him out to one of these trees, strip his clothes, and tie him to the tree naked. We call them punishment ants."

Deeper into the jungle, we come across a clearing where some sort of de-logging has taken place and the canopy of branches and leaves disappears to reveal the cosmos.

"Guys, can we turn off all the lights and just stand here in silence?" Guy asks.

We all click off our flashlights, tilt our heads back and stare up. The sounds of the animals fill our ears, the scents of the plants fill our noses, the bright stars fill our eyes, and the jungle fills our souls.

Sid asks how my stomach feels and offers me a mapacho. I decline the tobacco since I don't think it'll help. I put away my flashlight and decide to journey the rest of the trek in darkness to try to improve my night vision. My pupils grow as the distinction between objects becomes clearer: trees are obviously trees, vines obviously vines, and snakes obviously snakes. I hear a whistle behind me and watch as Victor turns and dashes toward the sound. Alipio climbs a tree like a monkey and hacks down a branch with his machete. The branch crashes to the jungle floor and Victor grabs a six-foot long viper coiled at its end. Lifting the serpent by the head, Victor calmly says, "This snake can kill you."

Sid, Guy, and Jon take pictures as Victor plays with the animal, seemingly akin to the creature as opposed to of a different species. Once we've had our fill, Victor instructs us to back away as he throws the viper off to the side. Unharmed, but startled, the snake sits still and waits for us to leave.

In the boat and en route to our jungle lodge, Jon and Tatyana talk about past lives and old souls. While the topics aren't foreign to me, the conviction with which Jon and Tatyana speak is. They're not theorizing about what they're saying, rather, they seem as certain of these topics as I am of the fact that I sit in a boat.

"A lot of people think there's a black hole at the center of our galaxies, but really, it's an intergalactic sun. Our Earth is ascending into that sun's wavelength, and a separation of the third dimension and the fifth dimension will soon occur. Souls that have ascended will join in the immortality of the fifth dimension, while souls that don't ascend will die with the physical Earth," Jon explains.

How do you know this? I wonder. *How can you say this with such certainty? What evidence do you have? Or, are you simply indoctrinated? Did you read this in some book and now you're convinced?*

I'm inclined to dismiss what Jon says, *but... what do I know?*

"Interesting," I say.

"Do you know about the fourth dimension?" Jon asks.

"Not by name," I reply.

"Well, the third dimension is this physical realm. This boat, our bodies, they exist in the third dimension, you know what I'm sayin'? Here, everything is external. Things happen to you. Occurrences are out of your control. When you move to the fourth dimension, you recognize that everything is internal, that everything in your life—the people, the events—are what you manifest. They're what you attract."

"Reality is what you make it," I suggest.

"Yes, you're in control of it. So, once you've reached the fourth dimension, you can ascend higher," Jon says, as I stare at him silently. "You know what I'm sayin'? I feel like I'm running my mouth."

"No man, you're not running your mouth. It's interesting."

We cruise along the still water, our vessel disrupting the glass river with soft waves. I shine my light at the passing shore and catch the eyes of a man fishing from a boat in the reeds.

We bank our boat and I run to the bathroom. The nastiness in my stomach has been brewing for nearly three hours and I'm approaching the breaking point. I kick off my boots, burst through the door, rip off my pants and sit down, barely making it to the toilet.

Exiting the washroom, I notice Carl shooing a large bug out of his backpack and I see a spider in our room's top left corner.

"Jon says some tripped out shit," I say to Sid and Carl. "It's weird. It's interesting. I don't think I believe it all, but…"

"I've heard him talking and I want to dive a little deeper, but he seems timid, like he's unsure about sharing," Sid says.

"Yeah. Well, true or untrue, his ideas are probably met with resistance a lot of the time," I suggest.

"Word."

Carl and Sid each climb into their beds. I tuck their mosquito nets under their mattresses for them before getting into my own bed.

Every forty-five minutes throughout the night, I drag myself from under the mosquito net and into the washroom to shit my insides out.

DECEMBER 29, 2013

The sounds of insects and birds crescendo as the sun peeks above the horizon like a child over a tabletop. I pop in my earbuds and listen to a guided meditation on abundance. *Abundance of shit*, I joke to myself before entering a tranquil space. My heartbeat slows, eyelids close, jaw slackens, and thoughts float by like birds in the sky, as I embrace the infinite energy of our universe and the infinite energy inside me.

After a twenty-minute meditation, I walk outside in my underwear and sink into a squat to open up my hips. I roll and twist my shoulders, spin my elbows, contort my neck, open and close my sternum, swing my torso side to side, and mobilize my hands, wrists, and ankles. I crawl around like a lizard, do rotational bridges, perform some pull-ups, and hold a few handstands before Victor announces, "Breakfast is ready."

We eat eggs and fruit before boarding the boat Alipio now drives. The trees ascend fifty, sixty, and some close to one hundred feet tall. The murky river water, which reflects a slightly overcast sky, splits opposing shorelines framed by thousands of shades of green and brown. It feels like a scene from *Apocalypse Now* or *Heart of Darkness* and I wouldn't be surprised if bows and arrows were aimed at our boat.

Breathing deeply, the rainforest air fills my lungs and refreshes my mind. I close my eyes and assume a meditative pose. *Joy, happiness, gratitude,* I breathe in. *Anxiety,* I breathe out. Over and over, I repeat the mantra, becoming relaxed and peaceful. The boat motor hums in the background as my counterparts chat.

Victor and Alipio find an entry point to their liking and bank the boat.

"What do you focus on while you meditate?" Jon asks me now that we're on land.

"It depends. On the boat, I was cultivating joy, happiness, and gratitude; while ridding myself of anxiety. Other times, I try to quiet my mind and watch thoughts pass. I've also done some of Deepak Chopra's guided meditations on destiny and I'm in the midst of another on abundance."

"Nice. Connecting with your higher self?"

"Umm, that's never a term I've used."

"Fair enough. Do you ever do group meditation?" he asks.

"Actually, group meditation in Koh Phagnan, Thailand was my first real exposure to meditation. I was there in 2011 and we did a variety of group meditations, including laughing meditations, which were hilarious. How about you?"

"Ah, that's so cool. Yeah, I do group meditations in Tampa. I love them."

Victor hacks some thick vines with his machete. His thrashings look destructive, but I'm sure he has a purpose. Vines in hand, he walks over to Carl, instructs him to open his mouth, and then vertically tilts a segmented section of vine. After a couple of seconds, a stream of water flows from the vine onto Carl's tongue. Carl takes the vine and holds it upright, continuing to drink from it for half a minute. Victor cuts a piece for Tatyana, Dan, Sid, Jon, Guy, me, and then one for himself. The water is crystal clear and tastes as clean as anything I've ever drunk.

"In the jungle, you never have to go thirsty, so long as you have a machete," Victor explains.

We trek deeper into the jungle. Plants dwarf our human statures and it seems like we've become miniature versions of ourselves.

* * *

March 1993, around the time of my sixth birthday, I'm at the *Honey, I Shrunk The Kids* exhibit at Disney World in Florida with my mom. The exhibit features artificial flowers that are twenty feet tall, lily pads that are fifteen feet wide, and bumble bees bigger than humans flying above our heads.

"Mom, do you think there are any creatures bigger than people that look at us the way we look at insects?" I ask.

"There aren't any that I've seen, honey," she says.

"What if we can't see them?" I ask.

My mom kneels down. "Well then, I wouldn't know. But sweetie, there is an awful lot of space in the universe. Maybe there are creatures bigger than us out there," she says, as she points to the sky.

* * *

Carl, Sid, and I lead the way and come across a gigantic tree with a trunk about twelve feet wide. Vines wrap around the old and beautiful tree, and the three of us climb partway up its base. We strike some cheesy poses as Tatyana takes pictures. We then ask Alipio to snap a few pictures of our whole group playing on the tree as Dan swings on a vine in front. We hope it will make a great promotional shot for Pulse Tours.

Walking along a path, I notice hundreds of tiny leaves moving across the ground in our direction. I wonder if these are leaf insects before realizing the leaves are being carried by ants. In the opposite direction, other ants march without leaves. I follow the slightly impacted path—a human wrist-width path sunken two centimeters below the surrounding dirt—for ten minutes. It's an ant superhighway! Tens of thousands of ants carry leaves in one direction while tens of thousands of ants head in the opposite direction to collect more leaves. The leaf-carrying ants disappear into a mound the size of a small submarine as leafless ants exit it. I imagine the series of intricate pathways, highways, arteries, and veins inside the subterranean ant city-state. I'm struck with awe and a subtle sense of fear, the same feeling I get when I stare at photographs from space that show our planet as a blue spec of dust. There is no ant with a hardhat and clipboard directing the others. These ants just *know* what to do: a collective consciousness, some divine design governing what needs to be done.

"You know, there's this story," Victor says to Sid and me, "that inside those mounds lives a giant worm. It's a worm that the ants feed, and in some way, the worm offers something to the ants. Maybe its pheromones or something, you know? It's sort of a…" Victor pauses to think of the word, "… a myth. I never believed it. I had never seen it in person. I had never seen it in any books. I had never seen any pictures. But I kept hearing about it. So, one day, Alipio and I found a mound and smoked it out. We filled one of the entrances with smoke and thousands and thousands of ants ran out. After a while, the ants stopped coming out. None remained inside, and many seconds passed. Then, a giant worm, thick and bigger than this," Victor extends his arms at his sides, "slithers out of the mound. The myth is true, my friends. The worm is real."

"Whoa!" Carl yells. Up ahead, he has dodged a black scorpion that hangs from a branch.

Carl has a dead black scorpion hanging in his bedroom back in Toronto, and he has just come face-to-face with a lethal live one.

"That's your most near-death experience, Mamma." Sid laughs. "And at the hands of your spirit animal!"

I learn that Carl can't remember ever having had a near-death experience, but knowing the way his memory works (he forgets inessential details more than anyone else I've met), this tidbit doesn't surprise me.

Victor shoves the shavings of a whitish plant under my nose. Garlic. "Eat some, my friend. It will help with your diarrhea," he suggests. I gulp some down and enjoy the taste. Victor places his hands filled with garlic under the others' noses and they all try a piece. Everyone except Carl. When Victor puts the garlic in Carl's face, Carl cringes and turns away. I wonder if he's a vampire.

We stumble upon some adorable bats nestled under big leaves, see more fire ants and insects, and then Victor explains that we're going to have heart of palm salad for lunch. Victor and Alipio give Carl and me their machetes and instruct us to cut down a palm tree. I stand on one side of the tree and swing the machete with my right arm, while Carl stands and swings on the opposite side. Having seen Victor chop a few different items with little difficulty, it's clear that neither Carl nor I possess the same skill. Swinging more than one hundred times and working up a sweat, Carl and I rotate around the tree and switch to our left arms. My first stroke is inaccurate, but I find my groove as we rhythmically slash the machetes against the tree, chunks of bark shooting off in the process. More than a hundred powerful swings with the left arm, and the tree begins to topple over. We move out of the way as the tall trunk timbers into a nearby tree and gets stuck up above. The prize heart of palm remains at the treetop, so Victor, Alipio, Sid, Carl, and I all grab near the base and heave.

"One, two, three, heave! One, two, three, heave! One more time. One, two, three, heave! One more. One, two, three, heave!" Seven or eight mighty heaves later, our tree disentangles from the other and crashes to the jungle floor.

"Jon, I want you to come over here and see how your veganism destroys wildlife," Guy jokes. Alipio hacks the heart of palm from the treetop and gives each of us a piece: an *amuse bouche* for later. Victor finds another section of vines and chops us each a piece for drinking water. Though I have two water bottles with me, I prefer to drink from the vine.

We walk along and Victor picks up a tennis ball-sized dark brown shell and cracks it open with his machete. Inside are white gummy creatures that look like maggots, but are in fact, grubs. Victor offers each of us one to try, and I'm quick to indulge. Biting down, the animal's insides explode inside my mouth and the flavor reminds me of coconut milk. Everyone except Jon eats one. I opt to have five. Each person makes a funny face as he or she bites into the grubs. Victor laughs at our reactions before he explains, "I could live in the jungle, so long as I have my machete. Without a machete, the jungle can be a difficult place."

We push through brush, jump over fallen trees, dodge swinging vines and thorns, cross small valleys over unsteady logs, and trot along open expanses when we come to them. Victor goes to a red tree and shaves off some of its bark before asking me to hold out my hands. He wrings the bark shavings like a soaked sponge and blood-colored juice oozes into my open palms.

"Drink that, my friend. It will help with your diarrhea," he says. I slurp the red liquid and laugh, realizing that I'd ingest just about anything Victor offers me. Though he seems to know his stuff: my stomach already feels better since he fed me the garlic.

He then grabs the leafy bark of a different tree, rips off seven pieces and bunches each of them into a ball. He shoves one of the balls into the inside of Sid's elbow and tells Sid to flex his bicep before sticking some of the bark into each of our elbows. Forty-five seconds later, Sid shouts, "Phew! That's hot!" and opens his arm to let the leaf fall to the floor. I feel a burning sensation, like a lighter's flame to my skin, and drop the leaf too. The others follow suit and release the leaves as the leaves become hot in their arms. Victor and Alipio laugh at their own prank.[6]

Victor smacks a tree trunk three times with the flat side of his machete as the sound echoes through the jungle. "If you are ever lost in the jungle, you swing and make that sound three times. It's like S.O.S.: you keep doing it and someone will come find you."

Trekking on, Victor comes across another plant. "This plant here is an antidote. If you're bit by a poisonous snake or spider, you eat as much of these leaves as you can and then rub the bite marks with the leaf. It will pull the venom from your blood."

We walk another fifty meters before I say to Sid, "Dude, we should grab some of those leaves and put them in my backpack, just in case."

"Good idea, Sandman!" Sid and I walk back and stare at the various plants in bewilderment.

"Do you have any idea which plant it is?" I ask.

"Hmm, I don't know, but unless we get the right one, this mission is useless. Let's ask Victor." We call Victor over and he comes to see what we're up to.

"Victor, we want some of those antidote leaves in case of emergency, but we can't tell the plants apart. Is it this one?" I ask, pointing to a plant that looks similar to the others surrounding it.

"Or, this one?" Sid asks pointing to another.

"No, no, no!" Victor laughs a deep belly laugh, pure joy in his eyes. "Can't you tell them apart!? It's this one," he says, and rips off some leaves that look virtually identical to the ones we had pointed out. I put the leaves in my backpack as Sid and I laugh, appreciating how badly we might struggle if we were left out here alone.

---

6   Victor later tells us that the leafy bark was shaved from a Chiric Sanango tree, often called a "fever tree" because the bark works to calm fevers when ingested. It also causes a burning sensation when placed on sensitive areas of the skin.

"Oh man, is it this one!? Hahaha!" Victor laughs on.

Soon after, we come to an opening where rope-like green vines swing from the treetops seventy feet above. I climb up a vine and as Victor gives me a push, I swing through the air like Tarzan. I straddle my legs and descend the rope while hanging with one arm at a time. Sid ascends another vine and swings through the air, while Carl grabs onto another and inverts himself. Dan also goes for a vine flight, as does Victor. Alipio ascends twenty feet up a vine, and I can tell these guys grew up playing in this paradisiacal playground and not on Super Nintendo. We experiment with different positions, take multiple flights, and smile and laugh like children of the Amazon.

On the way back to our boat, rain starts in the distance. I put on my poncho, board the vessel, and stuff Sid's camera into my backpack for protection just before a torrential rain pours down from the clouds. The water droplets fall fast and furious, exploding as they hit our bodies. The insides of my boots accumulate puddles and so does our vessel's floor. Alipio uses a pail to scoop water overboard while simultaneously driving us down the river. I remove my hood, look upward, and let the skies soak my head. Tatyana laughs and the others smile as we appreciate why this place is called a rainforest.

After a lunch, complete with delicious heart of palm salad, and a nap, we hop back into our boat en route to a nearby village to search for three-toed sloths.

On the way, Alipio stops the boat and we jump into the river for a swim. A bit groggy from my afternoon snooze, the water refreshes me as sunbeams caress the soft ripples on the river's surface.

At the village, we're greeted by a black and white dog named Emilio, who takes an instant liking to Sid. Carl offers to carry my backpack since the straps agitate an anti-malaria-pill-provoked sunburn I've developed. We walk past a number of smiling locals and a school that is out of session on this sunny Sunday. Carl swings a log around as though it's a sword and three young boys run through us playing tag. The alpha boy pushes Carl and runs away laughing.

"Hey, you can't just push me and run away. Come back here!" Carl shouts, and the boy returns with a mischievous grin. Carl and the boy engage in a joking duel in which the kid tries to steal Carl's log, but in grabbing onto it, is lifted overhead by his much larger opponent. The other two boys laugh as the alpha smiles in defeat, dangling from the log pressed above Carl's head.

"Mamma and her kids, eh?" Sid says to me and smiles.

Victor leads us into a field of high grass and tells us to pay attention to the trees. Alipio is nowhere in sight. We learn that Alipio and Victor have challenged one another. Whoever finds a sloth first makes the other climb the tree to retrieve the animal. Keeping an eye out, neither Dan, Tatyana, Jon, Carl, Sid, Guy, nor I see any movement in the trees, and I don't think Sid's new best friend, Emilio, pays much attention.

"I think I'm going to bring Emilio back to Toronto," Sid says, and I know he's serious.

Victor whistles to simulate the sound of an eagle—a predator to the sloth—in hopes of forcing a sloth to move and retreat from a tree. Fifty feet above, a sloth glides from branch to branch, swinging its legs with slow and controlled power, the most beautifully moving creature I've seen. Alipio appears and climbs halfway up the tree like Mowgli from *The Jungle Book*—two hands and both feet shooting upwards and grabbing at the same time. He gets to the branch where the sloth dances and leans out onto it. The branch won't support Alipio's weight, and with a bit of encouragement from us, he comes back down without risking injury.

We trod further to another tree where a couple of sloths glide up above, but it's too tall to climb. We then walk through a grassy area flooded up to Emilio's chin and hear the sounds of David Bowie's "*Major Tom*" playing from a building nearby. Four men dance and drink beer to an elaborate speaker system in a rudimentary bar. Sid and I bust a move and the men, obviously inebriated, laugh with us.

"4:00 pm on a Sunday: it's like one of our after parties back in Toronto," I joke to Sid.

"Yeah, and we've gotten past the dance music onto the oldies." He laughs.

Amongst the houses and out of the grasses, Victor appears with a furry and adorable three-toed sloth and hands me the animal. The sloth wraps its arms around my neck and plants its feet into my chest to embrace me. I stare into the animal's eyes, large black pupils vast and deep, and I feel a palpable love coming from the creature. I'm not sure if they're kidding, but Alipio and Victor talk about how sloths consume DMT[7] all day long, immersed in some psychedelic dream state; and I sense that this creature has an awareness of the universe beyond that of most others. I could hold onto the sloth forever, but I share him with my friends. The friendly animal hugs each member of our group, and then climbs on top of Sid's head for a photo op.

Heading back to the boat, I step in quicksand-like mud and my right leg is swallowed up to my thigh. I struggle to escape, pressing my hands into the earth and shifting my weight forward in an effort to not lose my entire body to the slime. I curl my toes as I wrestle free, but as my foot reaches ground level, I see that my flip-flop has vanished. I slide my arm into the quickly

---

7   Dimethyltryptamine (DMT) is a molecule found in nearly every living organism. Under special conditions, DMT consumption yields a psychedelic experience.

disappearing hole where my leg once was and feel around the mud. Dan and Carl kneel down next to me, all of us maneuvering our arms through the slimy stew, up to our shoulders in sludge. Ten minutes of searching and I consider abandoning my footwear before Carl and I each grab hold of an end and together remove my flip-flop from the swallowing slime.

We say a sad goodbye to Emilio before the young dog watches us boat into the evening.

Back at the lodge, Sid and I sit in two of the hammocks as the sun sets and talk about some of the challenges he's facing with his family's distribution company. He's trying to determine the best way to manage employees, so he bounces some ideas off me.

"It's hard to find the right people," Sid says. "And, I struggle with my employees not coming up with solutions themselves. Like, when I look at a problem, I take action. Some of the guys, on the other hand, don't do anything."

"Well, I think it's important to understand that none of your employees have the same incentive as you do. It's your business. If your employees had the same passion for it, they'd likely start their own businesses," I suggest as Carl lies down in the third hammock.

"Yeah," says Sid and nods.

"How do you react when your employees don't behave in the way you would have liked them to?" I ask.

"That's something I need to work on. I become passive-aggressive. Instead of just speaking about the issue when it comes up, I often avoid the confrontation, and then I'm sure my discontent manifests itself in my attitude toward them later on."

Carl chimes in then. "You just gotta be open, man. Your employees will respect you a lot more when you're direct. With my sales team, whenever one of them does something that doesn't suit our goals, I invite them into my office immediately to discuss it and set the record straight."

Guy, Dan, and Victor enter the gazebo to join the pow-wow. Now, we're five compatriots trading experiences, lessons, advice, and insights, all in an effort to help Sid figure out the best way to run his business.

I leave the gazebo to do some one-arm pushups, lizard crawls, handstands, L-sits, pull-ups, squats, and other movements, and Carl and Sid join me to do their own workouts.

"Dinner is ready," Victor announces in the melodic accent that Carl, Sid and I have come to love. Our family of eight assembles to eat a rodent the locals call "jungle rat", along with avocado, tomatoes, and the last of our heart of palm salad. The jungle rat tastes like pork and the meal is delicious.

After dinner, we board our boat to hunt for caiman, a type of alligator. Few stars shine through the overcast sky as I chat with Guy about the environmental magazines he co-founded and edits, and his two sons. We talk about *I Wager That*, the peer-to-peer gaming startup I'm working on, and my role as vice president of an advertising agency, all the while shining our flashlights across the black water in hopes of coming across red eyes. Victor had told us that a caiman's eyes appear red when illuminated by lights.

"You're really into health and fitness, eh?" Guy asks.

"Yeah, movement and health are two of my biggest passions."

"I love the feeling of being in shape. I like working out, but unfortunately, I broke my leg earlier this year, and I'm only recently out of my cast." Guy points to his right shin. "I see you doing handstands and I've watched Carl do a couple of back flips. It's like I'm down here with Olympians. I watch you sink down into a squat or walk on the sides of your feet. Why do you do those things?"

"Well, a squat is a basic resting position," I respond, "but you'll notice that Westerners aren't particularly good at resting down there. In fact, many people can't even get into the position. That's primarily the result of desk jobs and people sitting in chairs. If you spend eight hours per day sitting, your hips get tighter, your glutes and abdominals become close to dormant. This dormancy continues when you're engaged in physical activity, so your lower back takes a beating, because it has to work all the time while your other muscles slack off. Lower back pain is so prevalent in North America for that reason. When you visit Southeast Asia, for example, you'll notice people eating meals, comfortably seated in a squat. There isn't much lower back pain over there. In terms of walking on the knife-edge of my feet, I put my body in compromised positions as a form of injury prevention. If my ankles are exposed to twisted positions in a progressive and controlled manner, I don't have to worry about spraining my ankle when I land awkwardly while playing basketball. My movement mentor, Ido Portal, taught me a lot of this stuff, and it works. When I was younger, my ankles were weak. Today, I can jump up and land forcefully on the knife-edge of my feet without a problem, a feat that would hospitalize the average person."

"Man, that's smart," Guy says. "I need to incorporate some injury prevention into my training. I'd love for you to send me some information when we're back home."

"Absolutely. I'm glad you're interested. Most people seem to think that health has to deteriorate with age, and they sort of just forfeit to that notion. The reality is, if you move, eat well and smile a lot, you can be extraordinary well into old age."

"I know some old guys who are in great health. Of course, they seem to be the ones who took care of themselves and were active throughout all their years," he says while shifting in his seat.

"For sure. Movement is essential to life. You know, culturally, we evolve so quickly. Technologically, we're unrecognizable from our ancestors only a couple of centuries ago, and yet humans have been operating on the same hardware for 200,000 years: our anatomy is virtually unchanged.

We're designed to move, and to move a lot. I think that the lack of movement associated with modernity is largely responsible for many of the mental illnesses people experience today. People sit at a chair all day and stare at a computer screen, never getting much sun, and then their hormones go all out of whack, and they become depressed. Instead of teaching them how to move and live a life aligned with their biology, we tend to prescribe anti-depressants and treat the symptoms, but never the cause. It's a shame.

Similarly, so many little boys express symptoms of ADD and ADHD these days. Is it any wonder? They're so jacked up on sugary crap, and then forced to sit in a chair all day long to learn about some shit they're not interested in. Like prisoners, they get about forty-five minutes out in the yard to expend their energy, but the rest of the time, they're on lockdown. Restless, the kids can't pay attention, and then the school and the parents agree to prescribe the kids some Adderall and they think the problem is solved."

"Are you suggesting our culture is overmedicated, Mike?" says Guy, chuckling.

"Yeah." I laugh. "I guess it's pretty obvious that the current system is backwards, and yet most people pop some form of medication on a weekly basis, whether it's Advil or a prescription. I'm convinced that our hormones serve as signals, letting us know whether what we're doing is right or wrong. They shouldn't be so quickly suppressed with medication. They should be listened to."

The boat motor shuts off and Victor tells us to quiet down. Alipio pulls out a wooden plank and paddles quietly into some trees. I think they've spotted a caiman.

The three-quarter moon shines through the canopy above. Tropical leaves and vines dangle from branches. The trees' roots are submerged in the river with trunks ascending through the surface and into the night sky. The black water reflects moonlight as we drift further into the mangrove and I feel like I've been here before in a dream. Victor sits at the helm, peering into the abyss. He mimics frog noises while the rest of us sit quietly. The air has an eerie feel to it, almost like some predator lurks in the shadows.

"This is the perfect setting for a horror film. Maybe we're in one," Carl whispers.

Rain begins to fall in the distance and Alipio starts paddling backwards. Seconds later, the rain crashes down on our boat, flooding the vessel and our boots. Alipio ignites the engine and we head back to the jungle lodge through the nighttime rainstorm. Catching a caiman will have to wait.

DECEMBER 30, 2013

I wake up, meditate, move, and eat breakfast before we hop on our boat to a place Victor calls Monkey Island. Sitting behind Jon, I ask about the jewelry business he plans to launch.

"I love precious rocks and I love making them into jewelry for people. They have amazing healing properties, so I want to share that with people, and earn a living doing so," he explains.

"Very cool. Have you already started selling them?" I ask, skeptical about a rock having healing properties.

"Not yet. I think I'll start once I move to Hawaii. The energy there is incredible. The ocean and the volcanoes make it one of the best energetic places on Earth. Being there will really help with the creative process."

"Nice. I heard you talking about chakras the other day: the heart chakra, crown chakra, throat chakra, third eye chakra, and I'm sure I'm missing a few. They're not something I've ever looked into, but I wanted to ask you about the third eye chakra."

"Ok," Jon says with a smile.

"Linnea and I were making love a couple of weeks ago. When I looked at her, I saw a third eye between and above her normal eyes. When she looked at me, she saw the same." I point to my forehead above my nose. "I know seeing these third eyes could be attributed to the close proximity with which our faces were to one another and that we might have been slightly cross-eyed. I'm sure many would argue they were optical illusions. But man, it felt special. It felt different. We both felt a higher state of consciousness. And sure, some scientists would link that to the oxytocin and endorphin release associated with love making, but both she and I knew it was something beyond that scientific explanation. What do you think about it?"

"I think it's beautiful and real. The third eye has to do with higher realms of consciousness and clairvoyance. Is Linnea a Taurus?" Jon asks.

"Umm, her birthday is May 16th."

"So yeah, a Taurus," he says, laughing. "She's good for you, man. She'll ground you."

"You just guessed that she's a Taurus?"

"I had a feeling." He smiles.

"Well, you're right, she does ground me. I've learned a lot from her. Hey, we were talking about ascension the other day. Do you think it's possible to ascend without knowing the nomenclature?" I ask this in an attempt to uncover whether Jon's beliefs are those of indoctrination.

"You mean, ascend unconsciously? I think that would be tough."

"Well, no, not necessarily unconsciously, but simply without knowing the names of the different dimensions. In other words, could someone ascend without having read the books you've read?"

"Oh, absolutely. Ascension isn't reserved to one teacher," Jon assures me.

"Cool. So, you talked about ascending into dimensions beyond the fourth and fifth. What do you mean by that?"

"Well, when you clear all your karma, you leave nothing but love. If you keep clearing and ascending, you ascend to higher, more loving dimensions, and your soul eventually ascends into a star. You become immortal."

Normally, I would think Jon's bat-shit crazy, but for some reason, I choose not to dismiss the idea of becoming a star.

"Interesting. And, you think being a vegan's required to ascend into a star?"

"I think it helps."

"But, why is it okay to kill plants and not animals? I gather that you think killing an animal accumulates karma, but do you really think a head of cauliflower wants to be ripped from the earth and eaten by you? Plants are life forms too, and I think drawing a line between plants and animals is arbitrary. Maybe you just can't understand the language of the cauliflower's scream when you sever its roots."

"Because all plants form one consciousness. When you pull a cauliflower, the overall plant consciousness survives. Animals, on the other hand, each have an individual consciousness. When you kill an animal, you kill the consciousness, and when you eat it, you're eating death," he answers.

"How do you know all plants form one consciousness? I could just as easily argue that when you eat a plant, you're eating death. Death is part of life, and eating both plants and animals sustains our lives," I say.

The boat pulls up to Monkey Island and Victor hands everyone on board a banana. We sit for a while as Victor and Alipio make monkey calls. A few minutes pass before I notice some leaves and branches rustling in the distance. Two monkeys—one brown, one black—swing through the trees toward us. Leaping from branch to branch, the monkeys fly through the air, sometimes missing their intended target, only to latch onto another branch and continue along their path. The black monkey, better known as a Spider Monkey, climbs aboard and accepts a banana from Victor. Eating the fruit and discarding the peel, the monkey walks away from Victor, hops onto the boat's edge, and then tries to steal a banana from Dan.

"Whoa, whoa little guy, this banana's for another monkey," Dan says.

The Spider Monkey then climbs into Tatyana's lap and takes from her the bottle of tea tree oil she was holding. Tatyana pets the monkey as he nestles into her embrace.

The brown monkey, a Cappuccin, hops aboard the boat, walks around, but refuses bananas from everyone. Victor continues with his monkey calls and we see another pair of monkeys fly through the trees: a large reddish-brown Howler Monkey carrying a small black one on its back. The duo arrives to our boat, says hello, but they also refuse the bananas. The Spider Monkey, still in Tatyana's lap, tries to break open the tea tree oil and Tatyana can't remove the bottle from the primate's grip. Another monkey approaches the boat, and refuses the bananas.

"I think the monkeys are, how do you say, on a cleanse. I've never seen it before, but every ninety days, they eat nothing but grass all day long and shit and vomit to clean out their insides," Victor says.

A reddish monkey about four feet tall wrestles with a large black monkey high above in the trees to our right. I call them over and they approach. Then, the black monkey grabs the reddish one's tail and the two start wrestling again before turning around to disappear deeper into the island.

A couple of anteater-like rodents called Coati—cousins to the raccoon—climb a tree in an attempt to get closer to our boat. Lacking the athleticism of the monkeys, the Coati get stuck twenty feet away. They stare hopelessly, wishing for a banana. Knowing the monkeys don't want our fruit, I throw the rodents my banana. The pair of creatures pull off the peel and share the fruit.

With some coaxing and struggle, Dan and Tatyana remove the tea tree oil from the Spider Monkey's grip and send the primate back to his island.

As we leave the island, Jon and I start talking again.

AYAHUASCA: AN EXECUTIVE'S ENLIGHTENMENT

"Do you know what love is?" Jon asks.

"Yeah. I see love as an exchange of value. A symbiosis, if you will."

"Hmm. I think love is about loving all things, to treat each and every thing and every one as a sovereign being that's free to make its own choices."

"Nice. I like that."

"You're growing a lot. You're on an evolving spiritual path," Jon tells me.

"You think so? I'm always evolving, but I've never considered myself spiritual."

"Really? What do you think is going on in all this? What do you think about the universe?" he asks, while glancing to the clear sky above.

"I believe in infinity. I think the universe, the multiverse is like a series of Russian dolls unto infinity—without beginning and without end."

Jon smiles.

"So, a lot of my peers are psychics. They're who I hang out with…" he says, as I think of tarot card-reading, jewel-clad, leathery-skinned old women sitting in store fronts charging people fifty dollars to tell them their future. My bullshit meter nearly redlines as Jon continues, "And they said that while in Peru, I'm going to have a profound spiritual experience with a male Pisces who has long hair."

"Whoa…" My skepticism recedes. "I've only recently grown my hair out. I had a buzzed head for almost seven years."

"Well, I have a book for you. It's on ascension, and I know you're the person I'm supposed to give it to."

"Okay. You were told you were supposed to give the book to me?"

"Yes."

"All right," I say, pretty confident that I *won't* read it. "I guess I'll take a look."

"I think you'll find it very teaching," Jon suggests. "It speaks about the spirits of higher dimensions and how to become immortal."

I sit quietly and glance between Jon and the plants along the shore.

"What do you think about all of this?" he asks.

"Umm…" I continue to glance and ponder for a couple of minutes before responding. "The way you speak is new to me. I'm not the kind of person who's compelled to supply an answer or develop a conclusion so quickly. Sometimes I just need to sit with an idea for a while before I formulate an opinion. Right now, I don't know what to think about it, but I am thinking about it."

Victor points toward the treetops on the left shoreline and Alipio steers the boat in that direction. As we disembark, Victor runs over to a forty-foot tall coconut tree and scales it at a speed I did not think humanly possible. When he reaches the top, a large green monster crashes to the earth ten feet away and charges in my direction toward the river. It's some sort of giant lizard and I jump out of its way. Sid also dodges the lizard before Dan drops to his knees and tackles the Green Iguana by its torso. Pinned down, the animal tries to wrestle loose, but Dan's positioning goes uncompromised until Alipio picks up the creature by its tail. Victor shouts something from the tree above, and when I look back, Alipio holds only the detached slithering tail in his right hand. The lizard has shed its rear limb and disappeared into the water, its tail twitching as though still alive.

"Well, there goes dinner," Dan mutters.

Walking up to us, Victor shouts something in Spanish and shakes his head at Alipio then turns my way with a disappointed look on his face.

"You never grab a lizard by the tail."

Following an afternoon nap at the lodge, we hop in our boat en route to a local village. Over the last couple of days, Sid has organized a soccer match between our group from North America and Victor with his Peruvian friends. On the line is jungle supremacy.

"Victor, when we win, you and your boys have to bow down to us and say: 'you are the kings of the jungle,'" Carl announces while mimicking Victor's accent.

"And if you win—which you won't—we'll buy you a case of beer or something," Sid adds. Victor chuckles in agreement.

At the village soccer field—a grassy space with a few potholes and patches of dirt—Jon plays goalkeeper for our team. Dan and I start on defense. Spencer, another American staying at our lodge, takes midfield. Carl and Sid play forward. Guy volunteers to referee, and Tatyana plays goalie for Victor and Alipio's team.

The barefoot game begins with a lot of neutral zone play and not many scoring chances, though it's evident that Victor and his friends have chemistry: their passes are crisp and they know how to find each other on the field. Our defense keeps the ball out of our net for the first few minutes before our opponents score two quick goals. Some nice footwork and passing by Spencer leads to a goal scored by Sid, cutting our deficit to one. Carl scores another to tie the game up. The Peruvians respond to take a 3-2 lead before Sid, and then Carl, each score to give us our first lead of the game, 4-3 going into halftime.

At the start of the second half, Sid goes down with a toe injury. He can barely walk, so we sub in Guy to play defense as I move up to forward. Victor and his friends continue with their crisp passing and tie the game up at four. Throughout the half, the Peruvians score four more and we only muster one, losing the game 8-5. Despite an exhausting and competitive match, the squads exchange hugs and smiles, and we make arrangements to buy their team two cases of beer.

That night, the moon illuminates the sky and our group ventures out for a second attempt at caiman hunting, while Tatyana hangs back at the lodge for some rest. With flashlights and headlamps, we shine the shores in search of red eyes, as Victor makes various noises in an attempt to lure one of the alligators. After half an hour of searching, we reach a mangrove and Alipio shuts off the motor. Victor encourages us to be quiet as he sits at the helm, sweeping his light from side to side, scanning the black water. I don't see any red eyes, but Victor seems like he's onto something.

As I shine my light into the trees on the right, Sid starts to laugh at the front of the boat.

"Victor's got a caiman!"

Our guide holds up a baby caiman about eight inches long with black eyes. We take turns holding the slippery reptile who's stiff with fear.

"Only Victor could find the smallest caiman in the Amazon," Guy jokes. Carl pretends to kiss the gator as Sid snaps a picture before passing it to me.

"None of this guy's homies are going to believe his story: 'I was swimming around when I saw a bright, white light. Suddenly, I was snatched from the water and sent flying through the air. These giant creatures that stood on two legs were holding me, inspecting me, passing me around and flashing lights in my eyes. There were five or eight of them and they each stared at me and made strange noises, and I thought they might kill me. They were communicating with one another, but I'm not sure what they were saying. After a few minutes, or maybe an hour, I don't know, they set me back in the water before their ship and lights made loud noises and disappeared,'" I say jokingly from the caiman's perspective. "Ah, the troubled life of an alien abductee."

As our alien ship makes its way to the lodge, the motor seizes. Alipio puts a flashlight in his mouth, spins the propeller on board and inspects the motor. He tells us he's not sure he can fix it without the proper tools.

"I guess we better paddle," someone says. I ask Alipio to hand me his paddle. He smiles sheepishly and offers a heavy wooden plank. Dan removes one of the wooden planks used for a seat and begins to paddle on the other side. Carl removes a seat from up front and paddles at the helm. With canoe paddles, this would be easy, but with awkward twenty-pound planks, navigating our vessel becomes a tiresome task. I try to appreciate the workout as my shoulders burn, but then I contemplate the distance back to our lodge. We're half an hour by motor, so who knows how long this will take?

Carl, Jon, Guy, Sid, Dan and I rotate positions to switch between resting and paddling while Victor and Alipio work on the motor. We paddle for ten minutes, and I accept that we're on an adventure, which is exactly why I came down to Peru.

Now paddling on my left side, we spot some lights and a large building—a series of huts much like our lodge—on the right shore. We bank our boat and Alipio runs inside to ask for some tools. While we wait, Victor pulls out a few green buds that resemble marijuana, but with a more floral scent.

"This is chiric sanango and it will get you fucking high," says our guide, laughing. "It's a bit like weed, but different." Sid unrolls a mapacho and uses the paper to spin up a jungle joint. Victor lights the spliff, inhales deeply, holds his breath, and then exhales. His face relaxes, he smiles and announces, "Welcome to my jungle." We all laugh.

Everyone takes four tokes each time around, and the joint circles the group three times. Everyone but me, that is. The aroma's fantastic, but with our first Ayahuasca ceremony happening tomorrow night, I'm not in the mood to smoke. Sid describes the high as better than any weed he's experienced—somewhat similar, but lighter and happier. Everyone giggles, joking around, pie-eyed, and I'm reminded of many hazy high school days.

The motor starts and we all cheer. Alipio had returned during our session and repaired the motor. Back to the lodge, we go!

Cruising beneath the moon and stars, Carl, Sid, and I shine our lights into the night sky and pretend to have a light-saber battle, sound effects and all. Carl starts to sing in a made up language, a bit operatic, but very peaceful and soothing.

"Dude, this is my favorite singing you've ever done," I tell Carl.

"Yeah? After I establish a fan base with my current music, I'll release a tripped out album in this fabricated language. I think it'll have eleven tracks. *Oooooooohhh mooooooollllllllooooo sooolllliooooo oooooollloooo whhyeeeeeooooollooo soooooolllloooo mooooolllllloooo,*" he sings.

"You can call it *Solo Molo.*"

"Yeah, and maybe I'll put you on the cover in a meditative pose."

"Number one on the charts for sure!" I laugh and join in singing with Carl, and then Sid joins in too.

At the lodge, we gather in the gazebo and Tatyana joins us. We relate the night's adventure to her before Sid rolls up another chiric sanango joint and the others pass it around.

"Man, this is the best group we've ever had," Victor smiles wide.

We talk about the Amazon and Sid asks about the most adventurous thing we could do, if we were to plan another trip down with Victor. We discuss a trip deep into the jungle, far removed from any civilization, only accessible by aircraft. An excursion during which we travel only with a hammock, mosquito net and backpack. We hunt for food and become one with the jungle. Jaguars and anacondas will be the rule and not the exception.

"Victor, does anything about the jungle ever scare you?" Sid asks.

"When I'm with you guys, no. But, when I'm alone, yes." Victor sits up in his hammock and begins to speak with a slow and spellbinding cadence. "The jungle is a special place and there are many things that most people do not understand about it. I'll tell you a story of my grandparents.

One day, my grandmother and grandfather were walking along the edge of the jungle. My grandmother had to pee, so my grandfather walked ahead to give her privacy. A few minutes later, my grandmother hadn't caught up, so my grandfather turned around to get her. But, he couldn't find her.

From my grandmother's perspective, when she finished peeing, she could not find my grandfather, so she walked a bit farther to find him. She walked for a while before she came to a swamp where a young girl was fishing near a lone house.

'Can you help me? I've lost my husband,' she asked the girl.

'Yes, sure. Don't worry. Help me catch these fish first. After that, we will find your husband,' the girl said.

So, my grandmother helped the girl fish, and then they brought the fish around the swamp and into the girl's house, which was surrounded by jungle. My grandmother and the girl chatted, cooked and ate fish, and saw friendly snakes and jaguars. She spent three hours with this girl.

From my grandfather's perspective, my grandmother was gone for much longer. He spent the whole day searching, going up and down the path, exploring the jungle, but he could not find her.

At dark, he went home, and came back the next morning. He brought friends with rifles and dogs to search. They spent all day, from the time the sun rose until it set, shouting and searching for my grandmother; but nothing. No trace. They came back to search a third day. All day they searched: dogs sniffing, men going in different directions, but there was no sign of my grandmother.

My grandfather was scared, so he went to see a witch doctor that night. The witch doctor made a Toé brew[8], did a ceremony, and had a vision of where my grandmother was. He saw her near a swamp, and the witch doctor told my grandfather how to get there.

The next morning, my grandfather, his friends and their dogs went back into the jungle. They spent ten hours trekking in one direction trying to find the swamp. Finally, they came across the body of water and they saw my grandmother on an island of sand in the middle of the swamp. She was naked and covered in leeches. The dark water was full of leeches, plus electric eels and caimans, so my grandfather and his friends had to build a raft to rescue her. There was no house, no human life anywhere near. When they got to her, she was screaming and flailing like a crazy person. She did not know my grandfather. She didn't recognize any of his friends. They had to tie her up and put her on the raft.

They brought her back to the witch doctor, who gave her medicine, but she was still crazy. My grandfather had to leave my grandmother with the witch doctor for a week. Finally, after seven days, my grandmother returned to normal. She recognized my grandfather again, but all she could remember of her disappearance was being with that girl, fishing and talking to friendly animals for three hours. Nobody knows how she got to that island all by herself. My grandmother does not know how to swim."

Everyone sits still, staring at Victor.

"My grandmother is not the only one to have met this young girl," he continues. "Many other people have had similar experiences, in all different parts of the Amazon. They say she is a spirit who protects the jungle."

---

8   Toé, also known as "Evil Daughter" or "The Witchcraft Plant", is a teaching plant used by experienced shamans. For the inexperienced, the plant is potentially very dangerous and can cause delirium and insanity.

"What about you, Victor? Have you met the spirit?" Sid asks.

"I have not met the girl. But, when I've been alone in the jungle, I've heard whispers talking straight into my ear. Whispers of warning, not fun ones, and they come from a short, fat male spirit with one leg longer than the other. They call him Chullachaqui."

"Were you smoking chiric sanango at the time, Victor?" Dan jokes.

"No, my friend, no chiric sanango." Victor laughs. "They say Chullachaqui is a protector of the Amazon as well. Alipio has seen him." Alipio nods as Victor carries on. "Other people I've taken into the jungle know him too. There have been times when groups accuse me of playing tricks on them, making sounds and stuff. But, it wasn't me. Chullachaqui transforms into many different animals or even human beings. It may have been him who my grandmother saw as the girl. He's known to confuse people and make them disappear into the jungle. But, he is not evil. He's simply protecting the Amazon… the jungle is a special place, and there are many things most people do not understand about it."

DECEMBER 31, 2013

The jungle symphony begins as the sun rises in the blue morning sky. I insert my earbuds and press play on a meditation about abundance. With each breath, my body relaxes more deeply and my mind clears. My sense of self dissipates as I become one with all things. I am in the jungle, grounded with Mother Nature, and I have never been so at peace.

We eat our last breakfast at the lodge before we board the larger boat with our backpacks. I make myself a comfortable spot on the bench and lie down. Alipio steers us along the Amazon, and for the first time in Peru, I succumb to the temptation to listen to music. The groovy beat fills my head with colors as my feet tap and hips sway. Looking past the boat's edge, I watch as fluffy white clouds shift, expand, wisp and waffle, slide and gently roll in the beautifully blue sky. On the distant shore, brown trunks with green leaves reach for the sun and play in the azure at the same time a fish jumps.

Sid shares his iPod with Victor and our guide laughs and bobs his head to dance music he's hearing for the first time.

Carl sits to my left listening and singing to The Beatles' songs. His voice harmonizes with the deep house music filling my ears.

Guy sits smiling up front, across from him Jon lies staring into the heavens.

Dan and Tatyana sit in an embrace on the boat's bow, soaking up the sun.

I think of Jack Kerouac.

* * *

Summer holidays of 2005 are approaching; I am halfway through Jack Kerouac's *On The Road* for the second time. At 3:00 am, I close the book and call Carlyn, the girl who will become my first serious lover.

"Let's go to Mexico," I say.

"Ok. When?" she says, laughing.

"Right now. I'll pick you up in twenty minutes."

I sneak down the stairs past the guestroom where my grandmother sleeps—she's taking care of my brother and me while our parents are out of town—and into the garage. I start my parents' minivan, hoping my grandma doesn't hear the engine as I pull out of the driveway.

At the end of Carlyn's road, she appears under a street lamp with a backpack on her shoulders and hops into the front seat.

"Hi," she says, smiling.

"Hi." I smile back.

"What are we going to do?"

"Adventure. And, we can write about it."

* * *

After a ninety-minute boat ride, we're now at the river's edge, hugging and thanking Alipio, and wishing him farewell. We move our bags and selves into a white van and get on the road. The driver puts on some bubbly Peruvian tunes as we cruise along the jungle-side, modest homes, huts, and shacks interspersed between trees.

Guy and I chat about psychedelics and quantum physics.

"At the subatomic level, all things are indistinguishable from one another. Just a bunch of particles that look the same," Guy says. "So, if you zoom in far enough, you observe no difference between you and me, or between this van and me, or between this van and the road. It's merely our subjective perspective that identifies different entities and categorizes them. So really, the way the world looks is a hallucination."

"Yeah, the separation or the separateness of things is a hallucination," I respond. "Aldous Huxley talked about this in *The Doors of Perception*. While on a mescaline trip, he perceived no separateness between different objects. He was in his living room and saw the table and chair as continuations of the same thing, the same oneness. He saw the couch, himself, all objects—inanimate and alive—as part of the oneness, and it was as though the mescaline lifted the veil on reality. I had a similar experience when I was sixteen—the first time I ate mushrooms. That sort of realization occurs every time I eat them, and it's within this paradigm of interconnectedness that I perceive the world on a daily basis."

"Reality is so subjective. What we see compared to what a snake sees differs substantially, and yet, we're both situated in the same physical space. Humans can only see one percent of the electromagnetic spectrum, which means we can't perceive ninety-nine percent of what happens around us all the time."

"And who knows if there are other spectrums we're entirely unaware of?" I ask.

"Good point."

"And think about the way we affect reality. Like, how did we get from twigs and rocks, the natural landscape of Earth, to having skyscrapers and the ability to communicate instantaneously face-to-face with a person on the opposite side of the planet!? We have ideas in our head and they somehow come to fruition in the physical world. A skyscraper originates as thought in someone's mind, and then a few years later, there's a gigantic building in the heart of a city!"

"The imagination is magic. Everything we create originates as thought. What if all things originate as thought? Our whole universe," Guy offers.

"Perhaps," I say. "My friend Jason came up with a brilliant quote when I was seventeen. He said, 'imagination is imprisonment in an endless cell.' It'd be tough to convince me that anything is impossible. So many things we take for granted today would have been impossible five hundred years ago. The Internet: all human knowledge accessible with the press of a button. That shit wasn't possible even thirty years ago! So, when someone today dismisses something as impossible, I think it'd be better said that that something is simply not possible *yet*."

"Agreed." Guy says, nodding. "A lot of people want to dismiss telepathy as being impossible. Rupert Sheldrake, who's an author and scientist, talks about memory and consciousness existing externally, outside the body—somewhat similar to Jung's collective unconscious. He talks about a concept called morphic resonance: a connection across time from past to present. The idea is that every species has a collective memory and members of the species inherit knowledge from the collective memory, independent of their individual life experiences. Morphic resonance could explain the survival instincts and intuition we seem to be born with. And, it's the idea—an idea supported by studies—that if a rat learns a new trick in London, it becomes easier for rats in New York to learn that trick, even though the New York rats have never been exposed to the trick. Maybe it's like some unlocking in their DNA."

"It could also explain why scientists working independently of one another often arrive at the same discovery. There's a whole Wikipedia page that lists these multiple independent discoveries.

Or, something like the sub-four minute mile. For centuries, it was thought that running a mile in under four minutes was physically impossible. But then, Roger Bannister broke through the barrier. Two months later, two other men ran in under four minutes; and today, you have to be able to run a mile in less than four minutes just to compete in the sport. It's like a collective unconscious evolution of the species."

"And yet, mainstream scientists so often dismiss Sheldrake's theories for pseudoscience. Science has become so dogmatic that it seems less about open-mindedness and more about confirmation bias. In a culture that teaches us to be proud of what we know and ashamed of our ignorance, many scientists are uninterested in disproving their theories, and instead just look for ways to confirm what they think they already know. They're afraid to look foolish, so they toe the line instead."

"Well, I guess it depends where you look," I say. "There are lots of explorative scientists, but perhaps they don't receive as much widespread attention until years later. Science is merely a paradigm that tries to explain reality. Science itself is not reality; it is an approximation, at best. I mean, so many scientific theories throughout history have now been dismissed as incorrect. We used to know that the world was flat; we used to know that Earth was the center of the universe; and we used to know that Pluto was a planet! And, I'm sure many of the scientific theories we hold in high regard today will be dismissed in the future. Fringe scientists, though often ridiculed, are the ones pushing truth forward. Great new ideas are usually met with resistance. You can look at athletic coaches as an example. The best coaches are usually thirty years ahead of the evidence. They train their athletes using "unproven" methods and they don't care if there's no literature to back their methodologies, so long as their methodologies churn out world-class athletes. As for telepathy, I've experienced it first hand. No study's going to disprove its existence to me."

* * *

March 15, 2005, two nights before my eighteenth birthday, I'm on vacation in Daytona Beach with my best friend Kyle, his girlfriend Maggie, and our friend Kristen. The four of us find a hotel party with a bunch of seventeen to twenty-year-olds drinking beer and listening to music. Sitting at a table with a bunch of people we've just met, Kyle picks up a deck of cards.

"Sanders, I'm going to take a card from this deck and put it into your mind. Concentrate," he says.

"All right," I say, a bit buzzed. "Let's do it."

Kyle removes a card from the deck, conceals it so only he can see, and begins to stare at me. I close my eyes and see only darkness. I start to think of different cards: two of spades, three of hearts, four of clubs, but nothing resonates. I sit for forty-five seconds and can sense Kyle staring into my mind and the others around the table watching us. Suddenly, a visual of the seven of diamonds pulses in my head, almost like a headache. I open my eyes and say, "Seven of diamonds."

"Oooooohhh yessssss!!!!" Kyle throws the card face up onto the table and jumps up to hug me. "Fuck yes! I knew we could do it!"

"Holy shit, man." I hug him back. "That was so real!"

"Buuulllsshhiittt!" A few of the kids mock us, including Maggie and Kristen. "That's some sort of trick."

"I promise you, it's not," I say, indifferent to whether anyone else believes us or not.

"Do it again, then. This time, we'll be on the lookout for any signals," says the guy to my left.

"All right, we'll do it," Kyle says.

"Man, I don't even want to," I say to Kyle. "I don't care what anyone else thinks. I know that was real and so do you."

"Yeah, but I know we can do it again. C'mon…" Kyle pulls a card from the deck and again conceals it.

"I'll watch their legs to see if they're kicking each other or something," the guy to my left says, as he ducks beneath the table. Kyle begins to stare at me and I close my eyes.

I see nothing in my mind's eye, so I start to think of various cards, mentally scanning the deck: king of hearts, king of spades, king of clubs, king of diamonds, ace of hearts, ace of spades, but none of them resonate. I sit quietly, waiting for something to happen. Suddenly, the eight of diamonds pulses in my head, swelling and shrinking. I can see it!

"Eight of diamonds," I say, as I open my eyes.

"Oooooooohhhooohohohohoho!!" Kyle laughs and flips the card over to reveal the eight of diamonds. The others around the table yell and a few of them jump to their feet.

"Holy shit," I whisper. "Wow."

"Whoa. You guys didn't kick each other," the guy to my left says and extends his hand to take a look at the deck. Kyle hands him the deck, and after the guy inspects it for thirty seconds, he smiles and says, "I believe you."

"I don't," Maggie chimes in. "You guys probably practiced this routine."

"Yeah, you're signaling each other somehow," Kristen adds.

Yes, telepathically, I think.

"Maggie, are you serious?" Kyle asks. "You think we're putting on an act?"

"Well, I don't know. It seems pretty crazy," she says.

"If it's real, do it again," Kristen says.

"Sanders, do you want to do it again?" Kyle asks. "Let's do it, man. One more time."

"No, dude. For one, it's exhausting," I say. "Secondly, we know that was real. But if we're not able to do it again, then everyone's going to think I just made a couple of lucky guesses."

"I totally agree," a guy on the other side of the table comments. "You did it, and I can tell you know it. Who cares what everyone else wants to see?"

"Fuck that, man," someone else pipes up. "Do it again. Prove it."

"Sanders, one more time. The outcome doesn't matter. We've done it twice and we know that—nothing can take that away. But, you know we can do it one more time." Kyle stares at me.

"Fine," I agree. "One more."

Kyle removes a random card from the deck and conceals it like the two times before. He stares at me and I close my eyes. I can feel all the eyes in the room trying to find something to validate their doubts, but I don't care. I block everything else out and concentrate on trying to see a card in my head. I imagine some cards, scanning through the deck like the times before. I go through the different numbers and suits. A minute or a minute and a half goes by, and then the jack of diamonds is all I can see, all I can think about, like I'm in a dream standing in front of a human-sized card.

"Jack of diamonds," I say.

Kyle flips over the jack of diamonds and everyone yells and cheers. High-fives, hugs, and beer-chugging ensue.

A couple of weeks later and back in our hometown Strathroy, I'm hanging out at Kyle's parents' house with Kyle and our friends Hallsy, Spence, and Logan. Kyle and I relate the card-telepathy story in full detail to our friends over some drinks.

"Sounds pretty cool," Hallsy says.

"Bull-fucking-shit!" Logan shouts. "You guys pulled some trick and now you want us to believe it."

"Logan, are you kidding me? Have I ever lied to you?" Kyle asks.

"I don't think so, but you're screwing with me now," Logan answers.

"Show us," Spence says.

I don't know why I thought telling this story wouldn't lead to Kyle and me having to prove ourselves, but I did.

"Guys, I don't want to do it. It happened, and I don't need to do it again."

"Well, I guess we'll never get to see the great psychic abilities of Kyle and Sanders." Spence smirks.

"Sanders, let's do it, buddy. We've got this," Kyle says.

"I'd like to see it too," Hallsy adds.

"Argh. Fuck." I sigh. "Dude, I don't even know if I can do it right now."

"I know we can," Kyle says.

"Ok... fine, let's do it."

Kyle finds a deck of cards and before he grabs one, Logan takes the deck to inspect it, saying, "Have to make sure you guys aren't playing with a loaded deck."

Logan shuffles the cards before handing them back to Kyle. Kyle pulls a card and conceals it. He stares at me and I close my eyes. After about five seconds, the jack of spades fills my consciousness.

"Jack of spades," I say.

"Yesssss!!! Fuck yeah!" Kyle throws the card onto the table, face side up, and I jump up to hug him.

"Whoa," Hallsy says. "I'm sold."

Spence looks at me and smiles. "Wow."

"Are you guys kidding me!?" Logan laughs. "You're tricking us somehow. I have no idea how, but somehow. Do it again, so I can watch more carefully."

"Absolutely not." I chuckle. "I'm retiring from this game!"

"Sanders, let's do it!" Kyle says. "One more, just to show Logan."

"Dude, no way! There's nothing to gain. I know it's real, you know it's real. Everyone in Florida knows it's real. Hallsy and Spence know it's real. Who gives a shit about Logan?"

"Sanders, if I were you, I wouldn't do it. You guys know what you've done. I can tell you're genuine. No need to prove it over and over to everyone who asks," Spence says.

"Well, I'm not convinced at all," Logan says. "Unless you do it again, I won't believe you. I wasn't prepared that time. Let me watch more closely."

"I wouldn't mind seeing it again too," Hallsy says.

"One more time, man." Kyle looks at me.

"Dude, you might as well be singing vocals for Daft Punk. I don't want to do this forever," I say. "It's not easy!"

"I know, but, just one more time," Kyle says, smiling.

"All right, man… last time."

Logan shuffles the deck before Kyle pulls a card and conceals it. He stares at me as I close my eyes. Mentally, I go through the deck. I think of various cards and it looks like a small two of clubs lies on a vast black canvas. Though the card doesn't resonate like the previous four, I'm tempted to shout it out. But, I elect to think some more instead. Different cards float through my mind against the darkness. I scan through the deck—haphazardly at first, and to no avail. I start searching systematically: two of clubs, two of spades, two of diamonds, two of hearts, three of clubs, and so on. I spend three or so minutes with my eyes closed.

"I don't think I'm getting anything," I say.

"Just keep at it. I'm sending it," I hear Kyle reply.

I resume scanning, returning to a haphazard approach and focus carefully. Suddenly, the eight of spades throbs in my mind's eye.

"It's the eight of spades," I say.

"Hoooollllllyyy shhhiitttt!!" Kyle reveals the eight of spades and an eruption of cheers boom through his parents' living room as the five of us embrace like a hockey team that's just won the Stanley Cup. I run outside to go for a sprint around the house.

* * *

Guy and I continue our conversation for the better part of our hour-long van ride until we come to a stop where the paved road ends and a muddy one begins. Three moto-taxis and drivers sit waiting for our group. We hug and say farewell to Victor, thanking him for all that he's shown us.

Sid and I hop into the back of Marco-Antonio's vehicle, a friendly Peruvian in his mid-thirties, who loves driving his motorcycle and carting people around in the carriage it pulls. Carl and Guy hop in the second moto-taxi while Dan, Tatyana, and Jon take the third.

The terrain bumps, swells, rumbles, and grinds from the potholes and trenches that pock the muddy roadway. Marco-Antonio hits the throttle to plow through a deep divot. The engine redlines as the rear right wheel flies into the air and the moto-taxi tumbles to its left. Both Marco-Antonio and I shoot our left legs out and stomp them into the ground to stabilize the vehicle and prevent it from rolling. Marco-Antonio asks us to step out for a moment and apologizes for the inconvenience. With the load lightened, he rocks the moto-taxi backwards and hammers the throttle, the motorcycle and carriage weaving and sliding from side to side, slithering like a snake trying to escape the trench. Sid and I each grab a side and push as our driver steers and we break free onto smoother path again. We hop back in our seats, smile and laugh, and continue on our bumpy journey. We catch up to our friends in their moto-taxis and joke about this trip being like a Mario Kart race. I pretend to throw my green backpack like a green shell as we pass Carl and Guy, who remind us of Donkey Kong and Bowser, and Sid laughs like Wario. We shoot over a bridge that's five planks wide and missing its second and fourth planks, so that our tri-wheeled moto-taxi's front wheel rolls along the middle plank, while the back two wheels roll along the outside planks. If Marco-Antonio steers six inches to either side, the wheels will fall off the bridge, and so will we. But he drives cautiously and I'm confident in his abilities.

Over the bridge, we see a group of children and one woman swimming in a pond, and then Marco-Antonio points out a futuristic-looking building that turns out to be a university. I bounce in my seat and grip the roll cage tightly with my left hand, feeling grateful for my physical capabilities. I wouldn't want to subject my grandma to this ride, but I love it. We zoom along the winding and bumping road for over thirty minutes before we arrive at a gate guarded by two men with guns. Our driver waves to the men, who lift the gate as we proceed into the ceremonial grounds of Nihue Rao Spiritual Center.

The space is vast, with compacted white sand extending in all directions and forming a circle perhaps two or three hundred meters in diameter, the perimeter surrounded by jungle.

I hop out of the moto-taxi and walk along the sand past a large wood-framed dining hall with screens for walls and thatch roofing. The building next to it is similar in size, but with sturdy wooden planks for walls. Inside, I see a colorful lounge with couches, a hammock, board games, coffee table, and a library of books. I walk further through some trees and veer to my right past a concrete structure with four two-piece bathrooms on one side and four shower-sink combinations on the other. Past the bathrooms are our dwellings: a rectangular building, twelve meters in length, divided into four sections separated by wooden walls and equipped with screens for windows. Inside each room are two beds with fresh sheets and mosquito nets, a bookshelf, table, and a multi-colored hammock extending from one side to the other. Sid and I walk to the room furthest to the right. The number 8 adorns the door.

"I love the number 8. It's the infinity symbol tilted vertically," I say.

"You know, in numerology, the number 8 signifies financial prosperity," Tatyana tells me.

I'll take it. I set my backpack on the floor, get rid of my shirt, and head out the door to explore the grounds.

A path extends from beyond our dwellings and into the trees. I follow it for fifty steps and arrive at a small hut, large enough for a person or couple—a lovely place to rest amongst the jungle so green and the scents so fresh. I wander back along the path and Dan informs me that we're having a meeting in the *maloca,* and he points to a large, round ceremonial hut at the center of the grounds.

I walk through the open screen doors of the maloca into a space ten meters in diameter with a smooth wooden floor. Twenty-four evenly spaced-out mattresses with pillows are lined up around the circle's edge. I look up to see a coned roof of intricate and beautiful wooden architecture that extends about fifteen meters at its peak. A couple meters below the peak, a large, ten-spoke wagon wheel braces the coned roof. Three meters below the upper wagon wheel is a much larger wagon wheel with ten spokes bracing the roof at a wider point. Two-meter tall screens for windows connect the roof's base to a one-meter high wooden wall attached to the floor.

A soft breeze flows through the maloca as I notice a thin and agile young man with rasta hair and a young woman in flowing pants next to him. They are both shamans in training. Rafa, originally from Argentina and an American citizen, has been at Nihue Rao for two months, while Ana, hailing from Portugal, has been at the center for five.

I sit down on the mattress nearest the door and Jon sits on the mattress next to mine. Tatyana sits on the mattress to the right of Jon, then Dan, Sid, Carl, and Guy occupy the subsequent beds. With a big and warm smile, Ana sits down next to me with a clipboard. I extend my hand to shake hers, but she explains that she's on a particular plant dieta that requires her to refrain from human touch for a few weeks. She speaks slowly with love in her voice and eyes. Ana asks me questions about my health, whether I drink, do drugs or take medication, and whether I have any questions or concerns about tonight's ceremony. She thanks me for my answers then proceeds to ask the rest of the group the same questions.

A pleasant looking, short, bald Peruvian man with a sturdy build and heavy step enters the maloca and sits on the mattress beside Rafa. He is Ricardo Amaringo, Nihue Rao's master shaman. Erjomenes, another shaman, short and slim with deep dark eyes, sits down beside Ricardo. A short, round, and friendly-looking woman in brightly colored clothing then comes and sits beside Erjomenes. Her name is Ersilia. She is Ricardo's sister, and the third shaman who will guide us through tonight's ceremony.

Following introductions and a word about fasting at least six hours prior to the ceremony, we are invited one-by-one to share our intentions with the shamans. I sit cross-legged across from Ricardo and we exchange smiles. I speak my intention in English before Rafa translates to Spanish, and though I cannot speak Spanish, I know Rafa communicates every relevant detail. The others each share their intentions before we depart the maloca.

At 4:00 pm, buckets of water filled with fragrant flower petals wait for us near the jungle's edge on a bench beside the large fire pit where the Ayahuasca brew is prepared. I pick up a blue bucket and gently pour the water and flowers onto my head, then neck, shoulders, arms, hands, back, chest, stomach, butt, genitalia, legs and feet, covering every inch of my body. I rub the water and petals against my skin as I inhale the sweet aroma. The flower bath is designed to cleanse the mind, body and spirit, and to guard against negative energy entering before and during the ceremony. We're encouraged to let the petals dry onto our skin to enhance the protective properties and to make us more appealing to Mother Ayahuasca.

I look over at Sid and Carl, both covered in green leaves, and they each look like some combination of Tarzan, Adam, and a swamp creature. Goosebumps emerge from my skin, partly from the crisp refreshment of the bath, and partly from my excitement about tonight's Ayahuasca ceremony—an experience I've been looking forward to for two years; an experience I'm coming to understand as a rite of passage.

At 6:00 pm and minutes before sunset, Dan, Guy, Jon, Sid, Carl, and I head to the maloca to practice yoga. Rafa takes us through a yin yoga during which we hold postures for three minutes each. The practice is designed to relax and enhance receptiveness to the healing powers of Ayahuasca and the shamans. My breath deepens, my hips open, my body loosens and lightens, and my mind clears. As I enter corpse pose to conclude the class, rain pours through the jungle and thunder booms through the air. Through closed eyelids, I see flashes of lightning and listen to the showers pitter-patter the maloca's roof.

"Man, this is magical. The thunderstorm," Sid says softly, as we stand to roll up our mats.

"I know, man. Everything seems to be happening just as I would want it to," I say.

"A thunderstorm in the jungle on New Year's Eve, the night of our first Ayahuasca experience. Shit's about to get real!" Carl smiles and we all giggle.

I walk shirtless in the pouring rain back to my room to prepare for the ceremony, which begins in an hour's time. I'm mindful of each movement I make, appreciative of every breath I take, and I look around the room to determine what I want to bring with me to the ceremony. I change into the comfortable blue ceremonial pants and put on a grey tank top. I grab my water bottle, flashlight, a hoodie, and four mapachos, in case I'm inclined to smoke during the ceremony. Butterflies flutter in my stomach.

Around 7:30, I walk into the maloca and sit down on my mattress. A single candle illuminates the otherwise dark space. A happy excitement and lightness fills me and the air. I sit smiling as the others come to take their place. Jon bounces with giddiness on the mattress next to me as he and Tatyana share laughs.

"Mike, are you ready?" Jon asks with a beaming smile.

I chuckle, "Yes. How about you?"

"So ready. Enjoy the journey."

"You too, homie."

I glance around the room and everyone from our group is present.

Geoffrey, the man who participated in his first Ayahuasca experience with Dan earlier this year, and who is back at Nihue Rao for a five-week stay, sits on the mattress beside Dan's. A French man sits quietly on a mattress across the room. Ana, Rafa, Ricardo, Erjomenes and Ersilia are all here as well. Jon hands me a floral water that I'm to dab on my chest, back of my neck, both temples, between my brow, and on top of my head to protect against dark energies.

I'm called up first. Carefully, I stand. Striding slowly from my mattress and across the circle, my eyes focus on Erjomenes and the brew he pours into a small glass. I sit down cross-legged in front of the shaman.

Erjomenes hands me the glass of earthy Ayahuasca. I hold the reddish-brown liquid in my right hand, smell it, and whisper my intent to the divine spirit. I gulp the medicine, feel it slide down my throat and into my stomach. It tastes bitter, like a green shake without any fruit. Pausing a moment, I hand the glass back to the shaman, stand up, and walk back to my mattress with excitement in my mind and peace in my soul.

I am ready.

Sitting on my mattress with pillows pressed between my back and the wall of the maloca, I watch Jon, Tatyana, Dan, Geoffrey, Sid, Carl, Guy, and the French man drink the medicine. Rafa blows out the candle to create a pitch black environment before the shamans each drink their medicine and nausea brews in my gut—a nausea similar to that induced by other psychedelics: a comforting and teaching nausea, one that I know will persist, but will not trouble me.

Anticipating the trip and cognizant of tonight being New Year's Eve, I decide to reflect on my life lessons and experiences from 2013.

I reflect on my physicality—the incessant quest to improve my movement quality and athleticism—and how I became obsessed, training three-plus hours every day with a strict regimen and insufficient recovery, ultimately neglecting other areas of life essential to my happiness. I became constantly fatigued, exhausted no matter how much I slept. My strength plummeted, handstands became painfully difficult, and my body felt heavy, like I was slugging around anvils for legs. I would show up to work at the ad agency around noon and be spent four hours later. My energy had all but disappeared and the world seemed dark: both my sex drive and vigor vanished, and I finally resolved that putting a bullet in my brain was the best option if I couldn't feel normal again within two years.

Committed to overcoming the fatigue, I consulted with a natural health practitioner who helped me develop an appreciation for Yin energy, the female energy, and relaxation. I began a daily meditation practice, filled my mind with positive thoughts, and started to play rather than focus so wholeheartedly on the training regimen. This focus on play led to me eventually re-discovering the joy of movement and the reason I had become so interested in the first place. I could again use movement for fun—instead of like a drug that I needed a daily hit of just to feel alive. I practiced less, socialized more, and slowly but surely, became healthier and happier.

I contemplate the relationships I've developed and the people and businesses I've helped through my advertising agency.

I think about building *I Wager That (IWT)*, the startup I've been working on, and of traveling to the cottage of my business partner and friend, Charlie, where I first encountered the lovely Linnea. The way she looks, moves, her philosophies and energy are all things I love.

I think about traveling to Burning Man with Sid, and of experiencing the magic, the beauty, the people, the warm and loving souls, the music, the dancing, the recognition that this is what we live for—the existence that we ought to celebrate, and the infinite energy channeled from above that permeates all people and things participating. Burning Man is less a festival and more a way of life.

I think of my return to Toronto from Burning Man, so wonderfully uplifting. I am uplifted and uplifting to others. I think of how I developed a deeper appreciation for my expressiveness—through spoken word, written word, dance and movement, and through my ability to converse deeply.

I think of meeting Linnea at the corner of Ossington and Dundas Street, hugging hello, and then sharing dinner and rapturous conversation at Foxley before venturing to The Hunt Club gallery to see some of her magnificent art. The piece the name of which escapes me that now hangs on my wall: a grey, black and white rib cage with a belly full of beautifully blossoming pink flowers, makes me think that we are from the Earth like leaves growing on a tree, a philosophy of mine expressed visually by this woman I'm coming to know. I think of Linnea and our shared time together: rock climbing and meals. And conversations in which time vanishes: an intellectual fornication, the most oral of sex.

I think about the first meal I made for us: the ever-so-slightly overcooked bison liver, sweet potato/coconut oil/cinnamon mash, the asparagus, and garlic-butter roasted mushrooms, and red wine. Kissing her lips, her neck, and then stomach, a slight mental apprehension on her part—her physical readiness apparent—before she realizes that she can trust me with her whole heart and allows me to kiss, taste, and explore her with my mouth and tongue: a responsiveness and conversation so symbiotic that I become ragingly erect for the first time in a while.

I think about Linnea taking me in her mouth, the warmth and wetness so immersive, like my whole being is being caressed by her tongue. I enter her, a vessel into a port that feels like home. The cosmic rapture, the intertwining of physical and philosophical spirits, the orgasmic lust enveloped by love, the passion immersed in compassion, and the continually expanding vantage point into a reality and depth so profound.

I think about my Halloween trip to New York City with Sid to meet with some Burner, new and old friends; the *Robot Heart*[9] party of love, respect, and positive vibes with our fellow Torontonians, Art Department destroying the dance floor with powerful beats.

I think about the Burning Man book that Sid and I made, and then sharing it with Nala and Lara—two of the dear friends we made in the Nevada desert; the magical and immersive re-living of the experiences we together shared, an experience we will always have that cannot be taken away. This was a place of loving, emerging out of the sexual and into the platonic. The Sunday night with the four of us, plus our new friend, Enja. Half-naked, on mushrooms, and under the influence of entrancing music, we dance and share love in addition to a few drugs.

I think about my return to Toronto from New York and

---

9   Robot Heart is a collective of artists and entrepreneurs who tour the world spreading love and music with their incredible parties.

reconnecting with Linnea, our beings becoming increasingly intertwined. The verbal admission of love succeeding the ever-deepening physical and spiritual articulation of the same.

As I re-live my and Linnea's sexuality, I think of Mother Ayahuasca's desire for refrain from sexual release. I ask whether she'd be jealous of my mind's visions before recognizing that no, Mother Ayahuasca is attracted to this energy. But, I also recognize that the time is fast approaching to fully engage with the maternal root of the rainforest. Then, a fire rises and fills the right side of my body, the nausea mounting.

Instinctively, I say in my head, *Mother Ayahuasca, will you please wait a few more minutes as I reflect upon the rest of my year?* It's as though I'm broadcasting the thought telepathically.

I feel a presence, almost like a voice, respond, *Yes, my child. Take your time and let me know when you're ready,* and the fire recedes back down the right side of my body.

Holy shit, I'm talking with a plant...

I quickly and intensively reflect on *IWT*, the cryptocurrency[10] mining operation I'm a part of, my dearest friends, family and Christmas, then off to Peru where I'm warmly embraced by Dan, Tatyana, Jon, Guy, and our jungle leader, Victor. I think about my exploration, grounding, and integration with the Amazon River and rainforest, and I can feel that the integration is about to become more deeply rooted.

December 31, 2013 is the most peaceful day of my life, and instinctively, I communicate: *Mamma Ayahuasca, I am ready. I am ready to be shown whatever you would like and need to show me. I am open to any and all things, and I hope to learn from you, and I hope that you can learn from me. I welcome our collaboration, and I welcome you into me. My intentions are two-fold:*

---

10   Cryptocurrencies are emerging mediums of exchange, of which Bitcoin is the most well known.

1.) *To gain clarity on my business and career path: I Wager That is not yet where I had hoped it would be. Does this lack of success represent a fear I need to overcome—do I need to push harder? Or, is it an intuition I should listen to that suggests that I Wager That is not my right path?*

2.) *To gain deeper insight into my body: to learn how to recalibrate certain movement patterns so as to heal the neuromuscular pathways that sometimes manifest as discomfort in the left side of my body.*

With eyes closed, I sit cross-legged in a meditative pose, keeping the energy at a lower, less nauseating center, and I wonder if I'll vomit. I feel a series of warm visuals caress my third eye, my mind, my body, and my soul. Deep in the right side of my perceptual field and emerging from a distance, I see green and purple beams of light that remind me of Aurora Borealis. Like the Northern Lights, the beams flutter and wave as they slowly and lovingly reach toward me.

I open my eyes and transition into the physical world. The feeling of the beams persists at a slightly lower intensity, while my vision of them dampens to about one-fifth of what I can see with eyes shut. I turn my head to the left and can no longer see the beams. I turn my head back to the right, let my eyelids drop, and the visualizations return with the same rhythm as before, a little further on than where I had last seen them. These loving beams continue whether I consciously engage with them or not, the same way a cloud floats through the sky, independently of a viewer's gaze.

Everything that I'm seeing is objective.

The beams flow, waving and warm, and aim at my left shoulder. My concern for involuntary vomiting ceases. The beams turn my body so that I lie down on my left side and curl up in a position close to fetal. A warm blanket of green and purple Northern Lights envelops me as Mamma Ayahuasca shows me I'm safe.

There is nothing to worry about, my child. Relax, I will take care of you and everything will be all right, she communicates.

This is love, and this is maternity.

I giggle and sigh, and I wonder whether this will be the extent of my first experience. If so, that's fine by me. Just to have felt this warm and subtle embrace would be a wonderful and sufficient introduction. I think I might fall asleep…

A shaman begins to sing a powerful, melodic, and strange sound, not entirely pleasant, but far from unpleasant. Orange and yellow spots, triangles, and other shapes enter the left side of my perceptual field. The shapes move with the shaman's sound, emanating from his mouth and gently expanding rightward across my perceptual field. The colorful shapes seem to be forming a cloud-like entity.

Mamma is a portal allowing me to see and enter a new dimension.

Progressively, this new dimension takes the place of what was previously the empty space between my neck and the fifteen-meter tall ceiling of the maloca dome.

A second shaman's voice (Ricardo's, I believe) enters the dimension with red, purple, and green patterns. Ricardo's shapes dance to the rhythm of his song as they expand across my perceptual field before interacting with Erjomenes' orange and yellow shapes, combining to give the cloud-like entity more depth. Ersilia's song then fills the air with a full spectrum of sound and more colors than I've ever seen before—colors I didn't know exist, colors beyond the rainbow. All the shapes and sounds blend and fuse, and everything is untraditionally harmonious to my Western perspective. I giggle at the funny sounds and think about rolling onto my back.

Turning, I open my arms and heart as I feel Mamma Ayahuasca release me into this new dimension, a place I have never seen before. The purple and green beams of light gently sever from my body like an umbilical cord being cut, but she remains around me, in case I need support. Supportive, but not suffocating, the mark of a wonderful and loving mother.

I giggle some more and begin to hum to the sights, sounds, and feelings that fill this space and time, and still lying on my back, I start to dance, bobbing my head, shaking my legs, moving my torso, and gently pumping my arms. I feel like a five-year old skipping down the street. This is joy. Pure, unadulterated joy.

Three beings present themselves in my right perceptual field. Three small black humanoid beings cloaked with grey hoods and outlined by sharp and vibrant orange, pink and yellow lines.

What the…?

A bright orange line floats in the foreground between my head and body. A yellow line floats in the upper distance, while pink lines fill the background in an indistinct manner. The beings are female and about three feet tall. The one in front slowly reveals herself to me, opens her cloak, and sends me love. I wonder if Linnea would be upset by this encounter before recognizing that the being's expression of love is friendly, warm, protective, and maternal, not sexual.

The colors expand, all different colors flower and line my perceptual energy field amongst the loving darkness. I open my eyes to see whether this dimension is a hallucination. With eyes open, the visual of the dimension weakens softly while the energy remains present and accessible. I realize the dimension is not a hallucination, but ever-present.

By opening and closing my eyes, I can toggle between the physical reality and this new dimension; two dimensions that intersect harmoniously, but with a degree of separateness, like the way the air meets the ocean's surface. This space is unfamiliar to my conscious memories, but somehow familiar to my being, as though I've been here before. But, I can't place my finger on when.

I engage with the physical reality as I watch Sid light a mapacho. I look around the room and feel everyone's energy.

While I am on an individual quest, we are all interacting to engage with this space. The new dimension is differently present with my eyes open, and the film title *Eyes Wide Shut* resonates with me.

I close my eyelids to immerse myself in the new dimension some more. The three female beings show me more love as I hear Jon vomit beside me. I telepathically ask whether he's all right and I'm assured that he's just fine. I look at the female humanoids, and questioning what my eyes show me, I turn my eyes away and to the left, trying to test the spirits' existence. After thirty seconds spent looking away, the three spirits float over to the left side of my perceptual field, in front of my eyes and I feel them ask, "*Hey, don't you want to know us? Aren't you interested in what we have to share?*"

Hmm, I guess I'm interested in interacting with the beings of another dimension presenting themselves to me, I joke with myself.

I consider the communication that takes place in this dimension and realize that when the Ayahuasca or the spirits share an idea, they do so beyond words. Language is unnecessary and idea exchange requires no interpretation. The impartation is direct, nothing lost in translation.

I notice my own mind shifting between linguistic articulation of the experience and an articulation beyond words. I imagine trying to explain the feeling of falling in love to a friend with words. Unless he has experienced falling in love, my words will never do the experience justice. I then imagine being able to deposit my experience of falling in love into my friend's mind and into the fibers of his being. The latter is what communication is like in this dimension.

Caressing my soul, the three humanoid spirits shift further leftward and a new series of spirit species appear in the foreground.

I feel a sense of incompleteness and long for the humanoids, but receive assurance that they are always here for me.

The new spirits are each a series of six or seven worm-like tubes stacked on top of one another. They remind me of the inside of mitochondria, as depicted in my high school biology textbooks. I call them mitos. Unlike the humanoids, who remain floating in the background, the mitos have white eyes and glow with different colors: blue to black, yellow to black, red to black. With each colorful glow, my visual of the mitos' eyes succumbs to their soft, bright luminosity, like the sun shining behind a friend's face and blotting out her eyes. When the spirits fade to black, their bright white eyes become more apparent.

Then, the mitos turn brown and I see there are dozens of them. They grow and swell. Normally, I would describe them as disgusting, but in this moment, I see how beautiful they are and that they have a relationship with the brewing diarrhea I become conscious of in my large intestine. Eventually, I'll need to expel the diarrhea, yet I have full control of when that eventuality will occur. Now is not the time. I'm enjoying this new dimension too much to leave for the washroom.

My perceptual energy field becomes kaleidoscopic, but with less mirroring and more infinite in direction and potentiality. It is a kaleidoscope a blind man could see.

The mitos slide toward the background as a new friend emerges: a small male, elderly in love and wisdom, but youthful in energy and demeanor. He's as tall as the humanoids and has a relationship with them. He appears as a body propped up like a teddy bear's, with a horse's head. He is seated, legs in an open "V", with arms wide as though inviting a hug. His body is black with a vibrant and sharp pinkish-red outline. I sense his infinitely open and glowing heart, though I cannot see it. He shows without telling that he's a brother, a best friend, a grandfather. I think of him as Centurion.

The icaros[11] continue to vibrate throughout my entire reality, helping to shape it and see it all. I realize that without the icaros, perhaps none of what I'm seeing would be visible.

---

11   Icaros are the songs sung by shamans during Ayahuasca ceremonies. They claim to learn the songs from spirits.

I hear the percussive sounds of the beads on Jon's necklace colliding into one another as though they're centimeters from my right ear. I wonder if all these spirits are the ones Jon had spoken about earlier in our conversation on ascension, and I recognize that they are. Whether he perceives these spirits the same way I do or whether he uses the same nomenclature to describe them, I'm not sure, but it doesn't matter since both he and I are aware of their essence.

Initially, I was open to hearing Jon's philosophies, but maintained a healthy skepticism. This was partly because of the stigma attached to terms like "psychic" and "spirit", and phrases like "ascending to dimensions beyond the physical", but now I recognize the essence of what he articulated.

I confront the fact that our Western culture often criticizes psychics for not actually predicting the future and for thinking that psychics speak with vagueness and merely plant seeds that end up dictating the listener's experience.

While there are surely fraudulent psychics, I now realize that a "psychic" experience needn't be about prediction, but rather about guidance and helping a listener grow. It can be about helping a particular quest flower into all of its potential—a flowerishing[12] that transcends space and time. Thus, psychic guidance is a collaborative effort, much like my experience so far with Ayahuasca. A flowerishing much like the flowerishing of the Ayahuasca vine itself: a flowerishing that helps so many flowerish and flourish.

I toggle my awareness strongly toward the new dimension and see Centurion, seated and loving, still in the foreground but slightly less so. The humanoids have drifted closer than the mitos.

I begin to notice that my entire visual and energy field is made up of an infinite number of spirits, and spirit species, in a sort of

---

12   A word Rafa said that resonated with me.

sea that's navigable in a non-physical manner. In other words, the exploration of this spirit sea is beyond the third dimension and does not require my body, though I don't necessarily need to leave my body behind either. These spirits are all aware of one another in the same way that I'm aware of each of them. Biological, bacterial, humanoid, mammalian, serpents, plant-like, feather-like, infinite in degree and expressions, so many forms I don't yet have words to describe, and the more I peer, the more I see. Looking at the spirits is like looking in between stars in a rural night sky and beginning to see the stars beyond the stars. Every one of the spirits expresses love, each with a different articulation, collectively exhibiting love as a whole. I see love as the fabric of our universe, the creative force responsible for all things—responsible for the Big Bang and all its predecessors.

I am so safe and full of love and unbelievable wonder.

How will I share this? How can I express this experience? How can I articulate it to my own mind!? How can I integrate this experience with my previously conceived notions of reality? Will I paint it? Will I write it? Will I speak it? Will I produce a film? And will some who I share it with deem me insane? How!? What!? What the fuck!? Wow. Wow!

I giggle and sigh and *phew!*

It's okay, my child. You needn't figure it all out right now. You're being shown a lot, and you can simply observe for now, Ayahuasca communicates. *I'm taking great care to ensure you're able to integrate your experience later on.*

While these thoughts flow through me, the visual symphony of technicolor and spirits flows through my perceptual field. Peacefully, I lie back to enjoy the show as more beings appear and recede.

Enshrouded with love, I hear a whisper.

"Mike…" I look around and hear a second.

"Mike…" I inquire within.

Is this whisper a hallucination? Is it in my new dimension? In the physical realm?

I see the whisper present itself as small and energetic white spots of light in my left perceptual field. I watch the vibrations and navigate my body toward the source.

"Hey, who is that?" I ask aloud.

"Mike, hey man, how are you?" I think it's Rafa.

"Man... wow. Um, I'm amazing. I can't really see you..." I laugh. "Man, it's a bit tough to move, a bit tough to navigate physically, but wonderfully so."

I now realize it's Dan, not Rafa.

"Hahaha... awesome, buddy. Do you want a second dose?"

My mind explodes with a contemplation I did not realize existed. "A second dose!? Phew... no man, I think I'm good."

"All right brother. Enjoy." Dan smiles and walks away as I further contemplate a second dose, realizing that I am in the perfect place, in Mamma Ayahuasca's loving embrace. Another dose is unnecessary.

I sit up and stare with eyes closed, perceiving the infinity of this dimension, so grateful to experience this, comfortable with the idea of this journey either ending shortly or continuing forever.

I toggle back to the friendly spirits and notice the conversation taking place not only inter-species, intra-species, and with me, but also the species' interactions with my fellow humans in the physical world. I notice the soft glow of Tatyana's flashlight as her head intersects with the other dimension, the nearby spirits shifting to accommodate her presence. I smile and hum.

Rafa's white robe and energy emerge from my left.

"Mike, it's time for your song," he says, encouraging me to stand up.

I'm uncertain I want to shift my attention from the colorful spirits and am unconvinced the shamans can help further my understanding.

I better not go. Mamma Ayahuasca is and will continue showing me all I need to see. No human can enhance this experience.

But, wanting to respect the ceremony and feeling assured that I can always return to the new dimension in the event the shaman disappoints, I hear the Ayahuasca whisper: *Go. Explore.*

Feeling like I've landed on a planet with a different gravitational pull, I stand up and walk more like a two-year old than an adult. I stumble a couple of steps before finding my bearings as Rafa and I giggle our way to the shaman.

"Rafa man, this is magical."

"I'm glad you enjoy it," he says, smiling.

I carefully sit down cross-legged a few feet from some energy that I can't really see.

Disoriented in the physical space, I'm unsure if the shaman that sits across from me is Ricardo or Erjomenes. I stare at the form, which is about ten times larger than any human being, a gigantic grey and black swelling cloud of what looks like smoke. I have next to no idea where the shaman's physical form ends and his spiritual energy begins.

At the top of the cloud and ten-meters high, the spiritual energy begins to sway like a treetop in the wind. The sway slides down the cloud, building up steam along the way before it reaches one meter above the ground—presumably where the shaman's head resides—and the shaman begins to chant intense and mysterious melodies. I watch with dropped jaw. My shoulders slouch forward, eyes open wider than ever before—a new definition for awe. The song intensifies as more swaying, rotating, shifting, and waving emanate from the shaman's place in space. I laugh in disbelief, paradoxically believing it at the same time and sway in conversation and collaboration with this mighty form I behold.

Any other moment in my life, I would perceive this gigantic black and grey, bellowing and powerful form, inches from my face, as ominous and terrifying, but here, I am under maternal protection and I know this energy that sings and dances with me is breathtakingly beautiful.

The energy, the spirit, grows and becomes louder, sways more violently and comes extremely close. I want to touch the physical form but am unsure if it's appropriate, so I slowly offer my right arm into the energy field. We almost make contact and I wonder whether touching will be like sticking my arm into a soothing bath or a hellish fire, but I'm unafraid and confident in the former.

A giant burst of black energy like a mushroom cloud exploding from an atom bomb hurtles toward my face and five hands shoot from the cloud as two of them grip the crown and side of my head, firmly pulling upward as the cloud engulfs my skull.

I hear: PHOOOOOOSSSSSHHHH!!!

My head propels in the direction the hands pulled me as two more black bodiless hands explode from a group of five within the grey cloud, grip my crown and side of my head at a slightly different angle, and rip away in an intense massage-like manner.

PHOOOOOOSSSSSHHHH!!!

Inside this intense cloud of swaying energy like a tornado whipping me in nine different directions, five hands come at me again with two grabbing my neck and back of my head.

PHOOOOOOSSSSSHHHH!!!

Entranced in this exchange, I'm discombobulated and fearless. *What the hell is happening!?*

PHOOOOOOSSSSSHHHH!!!

Two more hands aggress my lower neck, tension slips away, I'm full of power, awe-inspired in a violent loving dance battle with no chance of damage. Surrounded by all-encompassing spirit energy, a cloud and five hands fly at my face; one grabs my left shoulder as another rips up my left rhomboid in the exact location I intended to heal with my second intention, and all tension vanishes. Complete muscular relaxation for the first time in three years.

The giant energy disappears, leaving only the slightest smoky trace. I thrash my head to the left and to the right, but the shaman is gone.

I sit still, unsure about what just happened. I peer into the darkness and through grey smoke I see Erjomenes sitting still as a statue far back on his mattress. His eyes are deep and intense, though I can't tell whether they're looking at me, through me, or to somewhere I'm unaware of.

"Mike, that's the end of your song," Rafa says as I regain my senses. I stand up in the most confused state and laugh in surrender. Rafa laughs with me all the way back to my mattress, where I collapse and whispering-yell, "WHAT THE FUCK!? WHAT THE FUCK!?. . . . . WHOOOAA!!. . . . . . WHAT. . . . .THE. . . . . FUCK!?. . . . . . WOW!. . . . . .WHAT!? WHAT!?. . . . . . WHAT THE FUCK!?"

I grab my head and shoot my hands up my face, over my crown and into space.

What!?. . . . . . What is going on?

I smile, mind blown somewhere into the distant cosmos, and I am ecstatic. Three tears fall from my right eye.

I become aware of the new dimension I've returned to and feel Centurion's love in the immediate background, as sideways serpents slither east and west, and then off into the distance. Brightly colored and slimy, these snakes would have previously frightened me, but here and now, they caress me with love. Full of beauty and soul, these snakes are not here to harm me.

I become conscious of my body existing both inside and outside this new dimension, the orange foregrounding line running across my neck, the dimension above looking like a pink and green Alex Grey painting. I perceive my digestive tract, intestines and all, full of different lively bacterial spirits. White amoeba-looking gut flora with eyes populate the space both above and below the orange line. Happy, Furby-like creatures are interspersed with the flora, and I understand my body as a vessel through which many spirits pass, physically living, dying, and being excreted; existences existing eternally.

My body is not my own, but a shared space for trillions of spirits—a universe unto itself—and I must continue to make this universe as welcoming as possible to the right kind of spirits: this to be achieved by continuing to nourish my body with all the right kinds of nutrients.

I feel the gut flora impart to me: *"a couple of things to help you welcome even more of the right kinds of spirits: stop eating dark chocolate and pork."* Before I can ask why, they show me memories of eating three squares of dark chocolate before every workout I did in the month of December, and that I was then only able to sleep five or six hours each of those nights. My attention shifts to pork. The gut flora and Ayahuasca show me memories of eating bacon, and that every time I felt a lethargy for the few hours following.

I hadn't been aware of either of these correlations until now.

Causations, my child, Mother Ayahuasca communicates.

But, I thought dark chocolate and pork were healthy?

They can be. But, they're not for you and your quest.

I recognize how important health is to me, and how my deepening intimacy with it facilitates the unlocking of my potential.

I ponder the feelings that make me feel best and most connected with my highest potential and my highest form of consciousness: love, gratitude, joy, peace, compassion, passion. I think about the people and things that help me achieve these feelings.

I think about Linnea as I become more attuned to Ersilia's icaros. Linnea's physical form appears briefly in my left perceptual field before she morphs into and reveals her spiritual self: a warm, glowing, slightly yellowish, gentle bright white slightly oval-shaped globe, reminiscent of a beautiful egg with a small black slit at the center, like that on top of a piggy-bank. I observe her energy for ten seconds. She is the warmest, most beautiful, loving, powerful, glowing, happy, pure, delightful, full-of-light, magical, wonderful, true, caring, lively, lovely spirit. Our souls embrace, merging together like puzzle pieces designed for one another and we glow radiant light. It is the most comforting, loving, and right feeling. It's the feeling of home. It's the feeling of being in my home amongst infinity. Our spirits express these sentiments together. This is a powerful and wonderful connection, one that values and protects one another's independence. There's an understanding that we needn't be together at all times, for we have our own individual quests, but that we are always connected and together in a spiritual sense and are always there for one another when needed. We both express *I am always here for you*. It is a support system of infinite depth made of infinite love.

Though I communicate with Linnea's spirit, I feel a compulsion to eventually communicate this experience with her in the physical world.

Is it even necessary to write her or call, or is she supremely aware of our spiritual intertwining of souls, despite my body being in Peru and hers back in Toronto on this final eve of 2013?

I know we will speak soon enough and I enjoy my time in her spirit's warm embrace. I could stay here forever, but out of respect for my personal Ayahuascan quest, she encourages me to *Go. Explore.* I kiss her goodbye and drift from the left side of my perceptual field along to the right.

I bump into my great friend, Simon. Our spirits hug with mutual admiration and we notice Centurion nearby. I see Ido Portal, a brilliant movement mentor, move from a one-arm handstand into a lizard crawl before transforming into an actual lizard. I see Ugis, the president of my advertising agency, who smiles and takes the shape of a big happy fish with glasses. The Ayahuasca, the shamans, and my concentration then guide my focus toward my first intention.

I contemplate my vice presidency at the ad agency. It's fun and rewarding, but not fulfilling enough to sustain me long-term. I look at the dimension of spirits and consciousness, all of it existing infinitely, consequential and full of profound significance.

This space is where I come from, where I was born out of, where I progress toward, where I dream, where my highest consciousness resides, and where I will forever and always be.

My vision shifts to the right, to what I have learned to be the more masculine side and see men dressed in suits who put on a façade in the name of business, all for a meaningless exchange of inconsequential information and money. Our physical world is merely transient, and those acts that do not contribute or connect to this infinite dimension and higher form of consciousness miss the point I crave to make.

So much of the business and governance that takes place in the Western world is driven by fear. These approaches are harmful and they make people unfulfilled and unhappy. The winner of the rat race is still a rat, and humanity's equilibrium has shifted too far into the masculine direction, thereby creating a fear-mongering patriarchy. The driven, goal-oriented, masculine Yang side of the equation is imperative to physical progress, while the maternal, present, feminine Yin side of the equation is imperative to spiritual growth. Only when man and nature balance in harmony will all have the potential for happiness and fulfillment. And, I feel called to help.

I stare into the realm of sentient beings to see an ethereal, white, porcelain-looking, hairless man burst head and shoulders upwards from a swamp. He punches his arms to the side and sheds his thick, shackled skin. He explodes upwards again from another of the same swamp, sheds more skin, and then explodes upwards again. The hairless porcelain man continues to ascend, again and again, ten times in total, punching his arms to the side and shedding more skin with each ascent.

From this vision, I realize that a lot of what I've been doing and working toward conflicts with my spirit and my true desires. I'm pursuing *IWT* due to my entrepreneurial yearning, and not because I'm passionate about the idea. It's a great idea, and probably one that will come to fruition—whether engineered by Charlie or someone else—but I am not passionate to execute the idea in the way it needs to be executed. If not for the money, which is a fear-based motive and not one emanating from love, there's no chance I would work on the project. If I don't admit my inadequate passion now, I risk putting myself in a position that will manifest in some ugly form a few months or years from now. And so, an honest conversation with Charlie needs to be had.

I think about my relationship with Linnea, as I'm sure my ambition is partly what attracts her to me. Though she's independent, I want to provide for us. But, I realize that if I operate from love, there's no reason to fear my financial future. I have no doubt about my ability to create wonderful and powerful things. What those things are, I don't yet know, but my creativity and time will help me sort them out. Is it writing? Podcasting? A combination of the two? A full execution of my love for full disclosure in an attempt to make the world a more honest, open, and loving place?

For now, I think I'll simply retract a little from my agency role and focus only on clients I have and the prospects whose values align with my own, all the while remaining open to other opportunities.

These thoughts live so clearly in this infinite and new dimensional space, yet my ego struggles to fully accept them. These revelations exist as realizations progressing toward, not as yet, foregone conclusions. The uncertainty does not scare me, for I feel Mamma Ayahuasca's whispering assurance: *Relax, my child. Everything will be all right.*

Beings and spirits continue to shift and drift like a mosaic of clouds in a big African sky. This is the most fascinating place I've ever seen. To think that all this exists and that I had no prior conscious awareness of it! Yet, it feels so right and familiar. I think of DMT, the "Spirit Molecule"[13] and the nickname is now obvious to me. This is the stuff we're made of.

I think of how I arrived here. I think of all my life, both physical and spiritual, leading up to this moment. I think of Dan and Pulse Tours bringing me here. I think of Tatyana's maternal warmth in helping Dan coordinate our plans and events throughout our time around the Peruvian Amazon. I think of Victor, our gracious jungle-guiding brother, a man connected with it all. I think of the shamans and Mother Ayahuasca showing me the portal into this omnipresent reality, the colors, the visuals, the feelings that continue to blow my mind.

I shift my attention to movement and notice the relaxed comfort in the left side of my upper back. I sense a message in the residual effects of Erjomenes' storm massage and tension release. I now have an intuitive sense for how to avoid the aggravation of old injuries: move more freely and always explore new forms and patterns. Work toward moving outside of and beyond patterns to a complete free form and flowing space. By not shifting and progressing from the same linear patterns, the same symptoms and neuromuscular expressions of ailment will re-surface. Believe passionately that my body is free to move in any capacity imaginable. Believe and act so passionately that this freedom becomes possible.

A giant flower emerges in the foreground. The flower's core glows a beautiful orange-yellow as its purple petals struggle to spread open wide, but it is covered by a white fuzz that inhibits

---

13   There's a fascinating documentary called *DMT: The Spirit Molecule* that explores the intersection of science and spirituality and of DMT being our link to the divine.

   DMT contributes to the psychedelic Ayahuasca experience. When orally ingested, DMT is not psychoactive for humans unless accompanied by a monoamine oxidase-inhibitor (MAO-inhibitor). The special preparation employed by shamans to brew the Banisteriopsis caapi vine with chacruna leaves containing DMT yields MAO-inhibiting harmala alkaloids, which render the DMT orally active.

the flower's maternal prowess. I see its core as a sun that gives the petals a fighting chance. Only if the flower receives a little more water and light will the petals free themselves from the fuzz and blossom into their full potential.

I recognize the flower as my mother and the white fuzz as the depression she has battled since I was a child, much more successfully in recent years. Her physical form appears. I am powerfully aware that all she needs to become truly happy is a little more love and a little more appreciation. With that, she will develop the self-love to blossom into the beautiful flower she truly is.

My mom drifts to the background as the physical form of my father appears in the foreground. He rotates as though on an axis, and I'm a bit unsure what to think or feel: a great and loving man, but whose spirit I cannot see. This isn't a bad thing, but I suspect he could be more emotionally vulnerable and open, which I speculate would allow for some personal growth. I want to ask him: "*Dad, are you willing to consider that everything you know about reality might be different than you think?*" I think about showing him Ayahuasca. As a physician specializing in internal medicine, I respect and admire his quest and ability to help people in suffering. Though I'm not sure his role needs to change, for he has helped tens of thousands of people, I wonder if a different perspective on the body, mind, and health as a whole could improve his practice.

I look at Western medicine and see it not as health care, but as sick care instead. Patients lead unhealthy lives for decades, and then look to another human being, and perhaps a series of green and blue pills, to cure them. But, health is not acquired in a day. It is built over a lifetime. The human body requires certain foundational elements to thrive: positive, happy thinking, sound nutrition, movement and physical activity, and a purpose: mind, body, and soul. No Zoloft prescription will ever provide those elements. In the Western world, we must evolve past treating symptoms to addressing causes. I'm confident such evolution is already taking shape and wonder if my dad could help it along its way.

Dance music emanates from a New Year's celebration in a village nearby. The music integrates with the icaros and I dance physically and spiritually with the tune. Centurion drifts to the foreground as pink and red fill the field. A large orange and blue bird flies to the forefront with a damaged wing. He flutters softly without direction and I can tell he's struggling to find one.

I recognize the bird as my younger brother, Rob, and I communicate to him: *I can help you mend this wing. We can do this together.* The bird smiles a confident smile. I think my brother would love and benefit from an Ayahuasca experience, allowing him to de-shackle from the chains he carries. Rob flies into the background as the humanoids and some new spirits appear together. I start wondering about *IWT* again as the friendly beings shower me with love.

One of the shamans vomits and Jon burps. Again, I hear the sounds from his necklace as though he's hovering right beside my ear. I wonder about the trip's conclusion and the brown biological diarrhea spirits float from beneath the foreground into the transitionary space between the physical world and the new dimension. I contemplate purging that which has been brewing.

I shift up onto my knees, locate my flashlight, and carefully plant my right heel onto the maloca's wooden floor. I press myself up slowly. It feels like I'm walking on the moon, my vision not entirely in sync with my eardrums and proprioception. I pull the door open and step outside in search of my flip-flops. Sid appears outside and his energy reminds me of a wide-eyed and happy lion.

"How are you, brother!?" he says and laughs. We exchange some "Phews!" and words of borderline disbelief before I leave for the washroom.

Inside the washroom, the new dimension is inaccessible. The maloca is a sacred space reserved for sacred exploration and this bathroom is reserved for purging, leaving things behind, and shedding shackles. I shit ferociously and with ease as I flash my light on the concrete floor. My bulb reveals faces that express negative emotions—emotions that have been purged in this room. I think of *IWT* as I continue to shit. I'm not sure if the new dimension will remain accessible upon my return to the maloca, but I'll be content either way.

On the toilet, I sit filled with questions and ponder like The Thinker. I take solace in the fact that a caterpillar does not become a butterfly in one day. Mamma Ayahuasca assures me that everything is all right now and that I am living my spiritual quest. It's never all figured out, but I always have my place in this infinite realm in which I have existed forever, and loving spirits all the time surround me.

As my body expels waste and toxins with the help of gut flora spirits, I receive confirmation that my digestive system is on point and that I should continue with the way I eat.

This moment represents the cleanest I've ever felt, and I recognize that my purges are not reactions to a poison, but to a medicine. I contemplate vomiting, but decide not tonight, and walk the twenty-five steps back to our ceremonial shrine.

Upon re-entry, a candle shines and the icaros have stopped. The ceremony ended during my purge, which seems fitting. I can no longer access the new dimension as I sit down on my mattress. Carl and Sid giggle, so I walk over to join them. Sid and I have more or less returned to sobriety, while Carl remains in a state of intense physicality. He focuses on gulping each and every breath.

"I…" He takes a big breath and continues, "have…" He pauses and gasps for air. "to think…" Another gasp. "about… every…" Big breath. "breath…" He gets the word out before giggling. "I can't… think… about… anything… else," he says brokenly, laughing again and rolling over onto his side.

Carl's intention for his first ceremony was to become more present. His mind often races and he wants to better appreciate each moment. Tonight, he can think about nothing more than the present moment as he purges through deep breathing and fluids from his nose and eyes. He had a second intention of learning how to better find the good in all people. He admits to being dismissive of new people when he becomes aware of a flaw in their character. He knows that something can be learned from everyone, so he wants to work on seeing past their flaws.

"Sid, what was your experience like?" I ask.

"Phew. Man, it was really positive. I had a lot of visuals and the prevailing colors were purple and green. The energy was very feminine; I guess that's Mother Ayahuasca," Sid explains. "There were all these species and animals on a lower plane that moved into this giant funnel that shot upwards." He moves his hands from out wide to inward, and then upward in a way that reminds me of a tree trunk rising into the sky. "It was powerful, unlike anything I've experienced before."

Carl reaches his left arm back toward us and feels around the mattress. "Guys…" He gasps for air before continuing, "even… though… I'm… not… talking…" Big breath and sigh. "I'm… still… here. You… guys… are G's."

"Thanks Ma. We know. You are too," I say, as I pat Carl on the back.

"You're a G, Ma," Sid adds.

"And Sid…" Carl gasps for air, "I know… I'm hard on you… sometimes…" He takes a huge breath. "sometimes the way… you behave… pisses me off… how you go… into Sods mode… and you'll bail… on commitments… you just… don't give… a fuck… but now…" Carl shifts around on his back and gulps for air. "now, I see that your mind… is like a work… of art… I've always…

understood… your mind… but now… I see it… as beautiful… I appreciate… it… it's like a work… of art."

Carl pulls his arm back and rolls onto his side as Sid and I smile at each other.

I relate my experience to Sid and we discuss how great a decision it was to venture down to Peru.

"Thank you so much for suggesting this trip, brother," I say with a smile.

"Thanks for agreeing to it, brother." Sid smiles back.

Fireworks sound in the not-too-distant village and Tatyana, Dan, and Jon light sparklers to celebrate the New Year.

Around 1:00 am, five hours since our journey commenced, everyone from the ceremony has either left for their room or drifted into a slumber inside our loving maloca. I lie on the same mattress as Sid to remain close to my brothers. I think of Centurion, Linnea, the humanoids, and Mother Ayahuasca as I fall to sleep.

JANUARY 1, 2014

I wake with the sense that it's 6:00 am, and according to my iPod, it is exactly 6:00 am. I head to breakfast and chat with Guy and Geoffrey before all of the night's participants meet in the maloca to share their experiences with the shamans and each other.

This group sharing is known as *conversacion*, and its purpose is for the shamans to provide verbal guidance regarding the previous and next ceremony, and so that they can learn how to guide us in future ceremonies.

Through Rafa's translations, Ricardo begins the conversacion by thanking us for being a part of last night's ceremony. He then turns the floor over to us.

Guy starts and explains that he had a fascinating visual and auditory experience. "I received some navigational tools for flying around this other dimension and my consciousness," he says. "Mostly, what I saw was intense and complicated geometric designs on a black or transparent background. I could toggle back and forth between this other level of reality and ordinary reality almost at will. The other aspect that made a significant impact on me was the singing of the icaros, particularly the female shaman's song, which for me, was accompanied by the singing of a celestial choir. It was like the shamans were creating the visions with their songs—literally singing the experience into existence."

Guy hadn't set an intention prior to the ceremony, but had simply been looking for an introduction to the sacred medicine, which he received. Rafa translates Guy's story for the shamans—as he does for all of the English speakers in the room—before giving Ricardo a chance to respond. He then translates the shaman's response into English.

Carl, Sid, and Geoffrey share what they each went through.

Tatyana then explains that last night's ceremony was her nineteenth. "At the beginning of the ceremony, I was surrounded by love and warmth. Everything around me was taking care of me, including a family of little creatures that I saw and connected with. They were loving, kind, and they reminded me of a local Peruvian family; except very, very tiny. I understood that I get what I give to others and that I am a very caring and loving person. I am a healer." She continues, "I asked: where does self love begin? The answer was: with self-respect, taking care of myself and having fun."

Going around the circle, Dan shares, and then Jon starts, "It was a really great and healing experience. I came down here for a cleanse and to strengthen my connection with myself. I actually threw up five times, which was great; I felt so much better afterwards. I had a number of visuals, some of which were confirmation for things I already felt, and others were scenes in which I was learning something new. So, I feel like everything was covered that I had asked for."

It's now my turn to share. I recount my experience with such passion and detail that after about five or six minutes, Rafa interjects, "Mike, I don't mean to be rude, but we have to keep it short."

I'm only about one-fifth through my experience, so I laugh and say, "I guess brevity isn't my virtue." Then, I quickly summarize the rest.

Rafa translates my story to Ricardo, though I get the sense that Ricardo doesn't need to hear the words and is already aware of everything I experienced. The shaman thanks me and everyone else for sharing before addressing the group with some guidance.

He speaks in Spanish, followed by Rafa's translation.

"We've had a special journey already. You've seen things you didn't previously know about, and the learning will continue. As we explore further, I want you to pay attention. I encourage you to sit up during the next ceremony and to be active in your journey. Keep your eyes open. Only lie down if you must. Focus on the icaros and your intentions. Mother Ayahuasca appreciates your active engagement. As you become more familiar with the medicine, you might discover new abilities. For example, you might be able to see the experiences the others in our group are having. You might see your friend having a difficult time and be inclined to help. Please be careful. By helping someone through their dark experience, you might absorb the energy of that experience. Since you're new to this realm, it might be difficult for you to get rid of that energy. At least for now, let us—Ersilia, Erjomenes and I—be the ones who help you through negative times. We have devoted our lives to understanding these realms and we have our own smaller ceremonies to purge the dark energy we absorb from people who take part in our larger ceremonies. There may come a time when you'd like to help others, but for now, all you have to do is focus on your own journey. If you do encounter any dark spirits, you can visualize a green net. Imagine wrapping the dark spirit in your green net, tying it at the top, and then sending it all away."

After conversacion, I walk to the art room to write. It is a beautiful mini-maloca-like structure filled with tables, paintbrushes, art supplies, and stunning Ayahuasca-inspired paintings and drawings throughout—so many of them reminding me of Pandora from the film, *Avatar*. The structure is made of wood with screen windows and is situated at the jungle's edge.

Immersed in rapturous conversation between mind and body, pen and paper, a little girl appears outside the most leftward window. She stares at me. I say, "Hola" and wave. The girl, probably four years old, looks at me for a few seconds longer, and then shows me her smile. She is beautiful. She walks to the second window then the third, fourth, fifth, sixth, and on, never once relinquishing her gaze. I glance down to my page and the girl presses on the screen to make sure that I know she's there. Telepathically, I whisper: *I know you're there*. With the jungle in the background, the beautiful Amazonian girl stares at me and smiles.

I spend hours channeling the first Ayahuasca experience to my journal. It feels like some celestial waterfall flows from the sky, into my mind and soul, out through my arm and into the pen, as words flow like water downstream onto the page.

Guy pops into the art maloca for an hour to do some writing of his own. He brings me a tea, but we refrain from talking. Carl shows up hours later, and after taking a glance around the room, he's inspired to paint: a dark, demonic illustration of black mountains and a large bird.

After the sun has set and with a cramping hand—it has been a long time since I wrote at length with pen and paper—I complete the story of my first ceremony. I make the final period and think: *I've got it*. As I close my journal, the Nihue Rao workers shut off the electricity in the art maloca for the night.

Walking to my room, Sid finds me and asks if I want to play Monopoly with him and Dan in the lounge. Not particularly interested in the board game itself, I agree to the opportunity to chat with my friends.

Dan and Sid set up the board and I gather apples and tea to consume while we play.

Early into the game, Sid takes the lead, executing deals and performing transactions with which I'm unfamiliar.

"I used to play with my dad growing up," he explains.

Guy arrives and takes a seat in the hammock to watch the action. I ask Dan about his intention during our group's first ceremony.

"Well, my intention was to cleanse obscurity and negative energies," Dan shares. "I also wanted a physical purge because I had been feeling a little blocked."

"Cool. Did it work?" I ask.

"Yes, yes it did. I had the best shit of my life." He laughs, as do the rest of us.

Sid builds a commanding lead as Dan and I fall behind. Barely able to keep my eyes open, I ask Guy if he wants to take my position. Guy agrees to the comeback attempt and relieves me of my duties. I walk to my bed and fall asleep before my head hits the pillow.

JANUARY 2, 2014

"Sandman, you want to go for a bath and swim?" Carl asks as I exit my room for the first time this morning. I grab a towel, and Carl and I take a fifteen-minute walk past Nihue Rao's gates down to the Amazon River.

We jump in and stand neck deep in the water, rotating in a circle about three meters apart from one another. The tall trees surround us while the calm surface of the water serves as both our eyes' horizon and floor. I feel part of the environment, not separate from it, as though I'm at home rather than visiting—as though I'm tapped into some eternal omnipresence beyond the transient physical forms.

"There's something powerful about the energy here, Mike," Carl says.

"I know."

"Man, your trip sounds so interesting. I want to see what you see, but at the same time, I'm not sure I need to. I think we're different."

"It was the most fascinating thing I've ever experienced," I say. "And you're right, we are different. The shamans say the Ayahuasca shows each person what he needs to be shown, regardless of what he thinks he should be shown. For you, I guess you needed that intense physical purge."

"I did. I feel so good and lean today, like something excess was shed. And apparently, you needed to be shown a bunch of beings that exist in other dimensions," Carl says with a smile.

We speak deeply and honestly for forty-five minutes before the conversation shifts to love.

"I feel like sometimes you're too quick to use the word love," Carl says.

"Why do you say that?"

"Well, I've seen you in three intense relationships now. With each girl, you've used the word love, and you've thought that you were going to spend the rest of your life with her."

"Yeah, well, that's because I've been in love three times," I say.

"Ok, maybe you've been in love three times, but I don't think it's possible to be *truly* in love more than once. For me, anyways, if I'm in *true* love, then I can't see how the relationship would end, barring death. There would be no reason to end a relationship based in *true* love. If you're truly in love with Linnea now, then I think the previous two relationships were lesser, and that they weren't true love."

"Have you been in love?" I ask.

"No. I've felt love for girls, but I haven't been *in* love."

"Well, I can tell you that I've been in love three times, and that the first two times were true. This time is definitely true too. People evolve, man. I'm not the same person I was when I was 20 or 24. When I was in those earlier relationships, I didn't see any reason for them to end. But, over time, and in both situations, I evolved and so did the woman I was with. And, we recognized that we no longer aligned. I still love both my ex-girlfriends, and though I'm not *in* love with them anymore, it doesn't make the experiences any less true."

"I respect that," Carl says. "I don't think I'll evolve out of love if it's pure and true though."

"Maybe you won't."

"For me, true love is infinite."

"For me, it's boundless, but it needn't last forever," I say. "Perhaps more importantly though, after seven years of friendship, I understand you better than ever before."

"Yeah, same. Or, vice versa... or whatever."

Carl and I emerge from the river covered in a thick brown slime, and though we came down here to bathe, the swim warrants a thirty-minute shower and the first real shampooing of my hair in six years.[14]

After changing into dry shorts, I venture to the dining hall. A beautiful spread of white fish, yuca, rice, beets, carrots, and peas sits on the table and I help myself to some of every option. Sitting down to eat, I notice that my relationship with food has changed and this simple lunch seems sacred. Each morsel bursts flavor onto my tongue, as I feel the nutrients travel down my digestive tract and integrate with my being. The transfer of energy, the fueling of my existence through food has never been so apparent. I have no desire to over consume—a far cry from my former self, who somewhat regularly lifted heavy weights only to justify a 4,000-calorie feast afterwards.

I finish my meal and head back toward my room where I see Jon standing outside.

"I saw the spirits you talked about!" I say to him.

"Yeah! You were pretty excited during conversacion." Jon laughs. "That's amazing. What did they look like?"

"They were infinite in number, but the ones I spent the most time with were the humanoids and Centurion. They all had black bodies; the humanoids had dark grey cloaks, and each spirit was outlined in the sharpest and most vibrant colors I've seen: red, pink,orange and yellow—like neon lights, but one thousand times brighter."

---

14   Up until recently, I had a buzzed head. Even with hair, I prefer to clean only with water.

"They had black bodies?"

"Yeah."

"Oh." Jon's cheeks sink and his smile disappears.

"No man, there's nothing to worry about: they showed me so much love!"

Sid walks toward us from the direction of Rafa's office.

"Hey brother, what's up?" I ask him.

"Man, just got back from a chat with Rafa. He's such a G. We talked about all sorts of stuff, and he's really helping me understand a few things."

"Yeah, Rafa's awesome. What did you guys talk about?"

"The biggest thing is that I'm trying to control my emotions. You know how I told you I become passive-aggressive with my employees sometimes?" I nod, and Sid continues, "Well, Rafa talked about how emotions are actually *in motion*. They're not really me, but instead, emotions pass through me, and that I should focus on observing my emotions rather than becoming them."

"That's a great way to put it," I say.

"Yeah, I really like that," Jon adds.

"So, I'm going to work on cultivating the outside observer within my own mind. He's going to send me some meditation resources. And Mike, I'd like to explore that with you, too. I know you meditate every day and I'd love to learn more."

"Absolutely, brother. Always happy to help."

I spend most of the afternoon walking the grounds and pondering in an ecstatic state. My mind has been opened to a new dimension and the knowing of this realm fills me with peace and a stillness that reminds me of a glass lake. The trees, plants, and sky are more beautiful than before and I'm more aware of the animals roaming through the jungle. I feel united with it all and sense the other dimensions and beings' presence, despite not being able to see them with my eyes.

I notice Ana walk into the lounge and head that way to talk.

"How are you, Ana?" I ask, as I sit on the couch beside the shaman-in-training.

"I'm good, Mike. How are you?" She smiles. "How are you feeling after your first Ayahuasca ceremony?"

"I feel incredible. Wonderful. For a long time, I've wanted to write a book and I spent all of yesterday writing. Articulating the Ayahuasca experience in words should have been one of the most challenging tasks I could possibly undertake, but the process was effortless and enjoyable. If the fifty pages in my journal aren't evidence that I should focus on writing, I'm not sure what is. And yet, I'm still a little uncertain about which direction to go in life, with respect to business and everything."

"Yes. It often takes time to sort out all the things you learn in ceremony. How does the uncertainty make you feel?" Ana asks in her Portuguese accent.

"It's interesting: I feel uncertain about the details, but very certain that I'll figure things out; so overall, I feel amazing about it," I say, and then ask, "You've been here for a while, Ana. Do you have any uncertainties?"

"Sure," she says. "But, like you, the uncertainties don't bother me. I continue to learn more from the plants—I also diet with plants other than Ayahuasca—and from myself each and every day. I won't be at Nihue Rao forever, and I trust that I'm headed in the right direction."

Just after 4:00 pm, I take my flower bath in preparation for tonight's ceremony.

During yoga, I struggle and feel irritable. Afterwards, I walk with Rafa to his office to chat and determine my intention for the second ceremony.

"As I'm sure you gathered during conversacion, Tuesday night was incredible. I gained a ton of insights, and honestly, it might have been the most profound experience of my life." Rafa nods as I continue, "But, even though I had so much clarity during the ceremony, my ego still doubts some of the revelations I came to. I've always wanted to be a writer, but I've suppressed it because I haven't known how to make a living from it. Two nights ago, I realized that I should walk away from my startup and just start writing; that's the first step. But today, I'm wondering: 'shouldn't I think about this more?'"

"Yeah, so it sounds like you have a bit of darkness to clear," Rafa suggests.

"Darkness?"

"Yes. Not so much as in evil—I really don't see you as a dark guy—but in terms of doubt and maybe a bit of fear. If you rid all your darkness, what remains is light, and you'll see your true path. You'll know what you're supposed to do."

"Cool. I also want to ask you about the spirits. Can you and the shamans see them, too?"

"Yes. In fact, you mentioned the Centaur during conversacion. You called him Centurion in your mind, I remember. I'm quite familiar with him," Rafa explains.

"Yeah man! He had this black body and was surrounded by a vibrant pink and red outline, and I could sense a gigantic heart! The humanoids were similar: black bodies with vibrant outlines!"

"So, those black-bodied beings are dark spirits. A lot of the shamans I've worked with, Ricardo included, suggest that those dark spirits seek to suck our energy. They're not necessarily bad or dangerous, but they're sort of lost souls, perhaps ancestors looking to feed off you."

"Hmm, but they were communicating with love."

"They can be pretty enticing. But, I'd encourage you to avoid the darkness and instead focus on the light spirits. An appropriate intention might be for you to focus on clearing darkness and opening your path. What do you think?"

"Seems perfect," I agree.

Exhale: *Clear My Darkness.* Inhale: *and Open My Path.* Exhale: *Clear My Darkness.* Inhale: *and Open My Path.* Exhale: *Clear My Darkness.* Inhale: *and Open My Path.*

Inside the candlelit maloca for our second ceremony, Erjomenes pours a small amount of Ayahuasca into the glass and looks at me for approval. Trusting his instinct, I nod, accept the glass in my hands, and speak to the vine, "Clear My Darkness and Open My Path. Welcome Mother Ayahuasca," and then bring the earthy liquid into my body.

Exhale: *Clear My Darkness.* Inhale: *and Open My Path.* Exhale: *Clear My Darkness.* Inhale: *and Open My Path.* Exhale: *Clear My Darkness.* Inhale: *and Open My Path.*

My eyes and head ache from repeating my intention hundreds of times. I feel tired already. Body warming, I remove my peacock tank top. I wait for the effects, confident that this trip will be unlike the last.

Sid vomits and I can feel his body convulsing. With open eyes, I stare toward the maloca's ceiling. To my right, I see two giant eyes spread seven meters apart. Forming an inverted trapezoid, two more subtle eyes sit five meters below the more pronounced pair and about four meters apart. The space between is black and void, so I perceive it as some sort of giant dark spirit. *I'm not interested in you*, I think, and close my eyes.

The icaros begin. A sense of boredom passes through me. Two nights ago, I was already enshrouded in warm, powerful purple and green maternal love by the time the shamans started singing. Tonight, I experience the subtlest of effects: mildly colorful visuals, only slightly more intense than lying in bed with eyes closed on any regular Thursday night. I don't think I drank enough.

I tap my feet to the rhythm of the beat and chuckle at the funny sounds. I hum softly and the soothing soft melody seems more like it's flowing through me than of my own creation.

Wanting to follow Ricardo's advice to actively engage with the icaros and my intention, I sit up and stare into the room. This lasts for only two minutes before I have to lie back down, exhausted. I yawn repeatedly as tears fall from my eyes one at a time. I turn onto my left shoulder and assume the fetal position. Immediately, a shit storm brews inside me and I leave to purge. On the toilet, I expel numerous bouts of diarrhea while I think about clearing my darkness. Dark faces and shapes swell on the candlelit floor, reminiscent of a mushroom trip. Much less pleasant than my first ceremony.

Back inside the maloca, I think, *I haven't drank enough.* I feel a bit sick, as though I'm coming down with the flu. I hear Ricardo vomit over and over, probably eight times in total, each time coughing up large amounts of phlegm, a very painful-sounding purge. I'm not sure I should consume more of the medicine, but I'm not really engaging with the plant. *I'm nowhere near the new dimension from my last ceremony.* I'm too much in my own head, in this physical space. I feel judgmental and irritable.

I stand up and Ana finds me.

"How are you, Mike?" she asks.

"Ana, can I have more Ayahuasca?" I ask with a slight sense of guilt, feeling a bit like I'm asking for more drugs.

"Yes, of course." She pours me an even tinier amount than my original dose. I imagine I'll have to come back for a third drink.

Tired, I lie on my bed and see only darker visuals with subtle purples and blues. While I'm not convinced the dark spirits I engaged with during my first ceremony were trying to steal my energy, I decide to follow Rafa's advice: I kindly ignore the dark energies and shift my attention elsewhere. I see little and the boredom and headache persist. I wonder whether my dismissal of darker visuals inhibits my trip.

Am I overcomplicating this? Last night was so much easier, when I engaged with everything and saw beauty in it all.

I take the fetal position on my left side and immediately have to purge. On the toilet, I focus on clearing my darkness. Everything aches, and I fold forward because it's too painful to sit straight. Feeling weak, I think about staying on the toilet for the rest of the night. *No, you need to work through this.* I then summon the strength to go back inside the maloca.

Back on my mattress, I'm exhausted, and the exhaustion frustrates me. I hope either something profound starts happening or that this ceremony will soon end so that I can just fall asleep and recover.

"Mike, would you like to come for your song?" Ana asks, as she kneels down beside my head.

Grabbing my bucket, I stand up and Ana walks me over to Erjomenes. Sitting across from the shaman, I struggle to make out his physical form, but only see a dark and grey energy where I know he sits.

Why do I know Erjomenes' black and grey energy is good, despite its color? Is there a chance I perceive light spirits as dark and that Rafa's guidance has misdirected me?

Erjomenes starts to sing and I feel his warmth. The energy sways while he sits, singing into his cupped hands. I gently sway in rhythm with his aura and song. I close my eyes then open them to see the shaman repeatedly raise his hands from low to skyward with open palms. A bubble starts at the base of my spine and rises up my navel, stomach, solar plexus, chest, and throat. My spine elongates, my head falls back, and jaw opens as a white energy beams from my core, through my mouth and up to the heavens, the sensation akin to orgasm.*Clearing darkness. Whoa.*

My head falls forward as my torso softly sways and the bubble begins again. Up from my spine's base, through my navel, stomach, and torso. My spine straightens, head falls back, jaw drops, and white light beams between me and the sky.

My head falls forward and I feel the bubble rise once more: up through my torso, as my head falls back, my mouth opens, and white light shoots from my soul to the sky. Head falls forward and back again, forward and back, each time with a gaping jaw and beaming energy running through me to up above.

The cycle accelerates and the whole thing feels wonderful and intense, but not feverish in pace. After seven to ten beams, my song ends. Amazed, I whisper "gracias" to Erjomenes before Ana takes me back to my bed.

Unable to remain seated for long, I lie down.

Clear My Darkness.

I feel a bit like I'm dreaming, about forty percent asleep, as I wonder about the meaning of Erjomenes' song.

What were those light beams of energy?

I sit back up to hear Ersilia deliver a song to Dan on the other side of the maloca. I love the way it sounds, a bit similar to the one delivered to me. A bubble starts beneath my naval and moves up my stomach, into my solar plexus and chest, my spine elongates, neck and jaw open, and my core and sky connect with white energy twice more.

Clear My Darkness.

I fall back to my pillow. Cold, I cover my body in a blanket and close my eyes.

* * *

A large whitish-yellow, fluffy and oozing cloud occupies a significant portion of my right perceptual field. A vertically-oriented green beam runs through the cloud.

How long was I away for?

I'm so relaxed and only half awake. I see my friend Sam, tall and beautiful, straddling the cloud.

I know what you mean about the place we go when we leave planet Earth. I've seen it!

This communication is a continuation of the conversation she and I had about her Ayahuasca experience some months prior.

"I know you have. It's wonderful, isn't it?" Sam smiles.

I'm mindful of Ersilia's icaros and, over my left shoulder, I see and feel the beautiful, warm, glowing, loving, lovely, positively-charged, yellowish-white egg-like spirit that I've come to know as Linnea's—the soul with which I'm united. We embrace and I am home in infinity once more. The encounter is brief and I float to the right to see more yellow and white shapes.

Whitish-yellow flowers twinkle across the lower third of my perceptual field. A green alligator with mouth wide open, bright white teeth, and pink serpent tongue starts eating the flowers as he slithers and rolls without travelling through space—like he's on some invisible treadmill. I'm unsure whether he's stealing my flowers or if he's helping me out, but he makes me slightly uncomfortable, so I tune him out.

I notice a light in the physical world and turn my head left. I see Ana walking another woman (*who is she?*) to a place four meters away where a mattress didn't previously lie. Ana walks away and I'm mesmerized by this new female human (*is she human?*), who sits upright and stares into the center of the maloca.

Who is she? Where did she come from?

She sits still and my gaze intensifies. I look away, turn my head back to center and feel an open portal—a liquid-like, translucent tube that reminds me of the large soap bubble portals depicted in *Donnie Darko*. On the left side of my head, it feels like the skin and bone open up, as a portal emanates from me and connects with the head of the woman to my left. Uncertain about her energy and realness (*is she a hallucination?*) and having earlier been taught that it's important to protect myself from others' energies, I try to close the portal. With conscious might, I shrink the hole a little, and then place my hand over the portal to interrupt its flow. I massage my head, thinking that I can rub it shut. After a few minutes, I feel the portal close, but some of the disturbance remains, like an open wound sewn shut. I wonder whether some spirit(s)—good or bad—crossed from her field to mine.

A series of purple lines wave amongst a black cloud and I imagine it to be a visitor from the woman's space. I'm inclined to engage, but respecting Rafa's advice, I pay the dark cloud no mind.

A yellow banana emerges from a white cream and it looks tasty. I'm so hungry and I want the ceremony to end. I gasp as though I've been startled—by what, I'm not sure; the same feeling of falling that occurs just before sleep, known as a hypnic jerk. Usually, when I experience a hypnic jerk before sleep, it's accompanied by a visual and a lapse in consciousness, but this gasp was accompanied by neither.

I yawn and yawn. I've never felt so physically drained. I want to sleep, and assume the fetal position, instantaneously having to purge. I find the strength to stand and hustle outside to shit in the toilet. These are flu-like symptoms. I'm not sure they're good. First ceremony, I never once thought of Ayahuasca as toxic. I saw it as a healing plant and medicine. Tonight, I wonder whether it's a poisonous drug, but I maintain focus on clearing my darkness. I'm confident the vine is clearing out spirits that have overstayed their welcome. I leave a reddish-brown mess in the bowl before I flush.

I struggle to find my mattress, and when I do, collapse onto the pillow and cover myself in the blanket. I'm cold, but unwilling to put on my peacock shirt; it doesn't feel right. I again gasp as though falling, a startling yet somehow enjoyable sensation, and I feel weak. But I'm compelled to sit upright, wanting to respect Ricardo's advice. I fight to maintain posture before falling onto my back.

* * *

I've been immersed in yellow and white for I don't know how long. I see a slithering snake, yellow with white spots, in my upper right perceptual field. I realize I've been half asleep before I see angels rise amongst white fluffy clouds in a crystal blue sky. The kinds of angels found on stained glass windows of Catholic churches; the kinds of angels I didn't believe to exist. One halo separates from its angel, as the other angels disappear. A bright spotlight shines on Carl in the physical space. He sits upright with legs extended in front of him, eyes closed with a stoic look on his face, and I see the once separate halo now floating and shining atop his head.

He is my angel and helps protect me.

Before now, I did not think this possible. One of my best friends, who I love and respect, but who has some behaviors and philosophies I oppose. I think back to the conversation we had in the slimy river earlier this morning. I've always trusted him, but now I trust him with my life. He is one of my guardians.

I think of Sid and see an empty halo floating in a bright blue sky before my shaggy-red-haired, lion-like friend rises through the clouds wearing a big smile. Sid merges with the halo, and I recognize that he too protects me—a guardian angel.

I sit up again to keep clearing my darkness and open my path.

Follow the light.

I fall back, yawn, shed tears, and gasp numerous times to the sensation of falling. I curl to my left, knowing I'll have to shit, and surely, I do. In the washroom, with my body folded forward to mitigate the pain, I wonder when the ceremony will end. Anytime now will do.

Upon return to my spot inside the maloca, I try to sit upright.

This world is so strange, the experience so exhausting, difficult without fear. Maybe this is exactly what I needed, and perhaps Rafa was right after all: my patience allowing me to see the light spirits he told me about some hours before.

Peace fills me, but not to the brim. I've progressed, but there remains darkness to clear and work to do. I contemplate life as a therapist and a writer, and how simple that would be: a service to both myself and to others, pure to my core. *IWT* is not for me.

A bright sun shines in the upper right field, its rays peering through dark forest trees. The sun wants to beam straight into my soul, and while it does a good job trying, some shadows remain. I use my energy to pull the trees out of the way as a few more sunrays warm my being. I feel like I'm physically uprooting giant oak trees and it's as laboring as I would imagine it to be in the physical world. I struggle to pull more as my consciousness fades.

* * *

The icaros have subsided and Ricardo and Erjomenes laugh in the middle of a song. Then, all three shamans chuckle with joy. I can tell they've cracked a joke about a certain female spirit's interpretation of our group and I sense that the spirit appreciates the comedy. The happiness warms me with love and I'm fascinated by my ability to believe what I'm experiencing.

The icaros end. The experience has been difficult, but good. I feel a song come through me as I hum a gentle tune. Soothing my heart and soul, I let the tune trail into the cosmos.

* * *

A single candlelight fills the maloca. I'm not sure how long I was gone for, but it feels like 2:00 am. Exhausted and barely able to move, I feel it essential for one last purge.

En route to the toilet, I look up at the stars: the beautifully ascended souls I now think them to be, and I cry a happy tear. I find a kitten and pet her with boundless love.

JANUARY 3, 2014

I gather my belongings and Sid, and we head to our room.

Inspired to write, I'm unable to sleep. I sit in bed with a headlamp, journal, and pen before moving outside when dawn arrives. A young yellow lab named Happy finds me sitting on a log. I pet and massage the dog. His energy is so pure, I love him so much, and he feels more like a brother than a pet.

For hours, Happy sits against my foot as I write and write until my hand gives out, at which time Sid comes to talk. He tells me about his second ceremony.

"Man, it was so difficult. I had a complete physical and psychological breakdown. I purged through my eyes, my nose, I vomited, I sweat, diarrhea; physically, it was rough. Mentally, it was further removed from sanity than I've ever been. I lost touch with reality. I was asking myself, 'Why am I in Peru? Am I in Peru? Why am I drinking Ayahuasca?'"

"Did you ever wonder if you might be lost forever?" I ask.

"That's the thing: I did have that thought, but I knew you, Carl, and Dan were here, and I knew that eventually I would return to reality," Sid says, his voice laced with exhaustion and gratitude.

The Ayahuasca is taking care of Sid, too.

In the dining hall, I end a twenty-one-hour fast with thirteen eggs, three sweet potatoes, a heaping scoop of rice, beets and carrots—each and every bite delicious and essential. While nourishing my body, Guy shares his experience.

"I entered the ceremony with the intent to work on my ability to have loving relationships," he starts. "Soon after the medicine took effect, I realized that it was my heart region that needed work. I laid down on what seemed like an operating table in this other reality, and the shamans were performing an operation on my heart, as though they were surgeons. They were working on removing all this phlegm, blockages, and gunk surrounding my heart center. It was exhausting. I was drifting in and out of consciousness, but I heard this voice: 'Stay awake. Pay attention. This is important. Keep breathing.' So, I fought to remain present. I was then instructed to sit up. When I did, I saw Ricardo vomiting enormous amounts of phlegm into his plastic bucket. It was a violent purge and he kept purging and purging, over and over again. I recognized that the phlegm he expelled were my blockages. Ricardo was doing the work and enduring this purge as a means to help me." Guy pauses as tears well in his eyes, and I assume he's being a bit self-absorbed to think Ricardo's powerful pukes were all about him. Guy continues, saying, "I can't be more grateful for the work these shamans do. They're like Olympic athletes. I'm going to thank Ricardo when I see him."

A North American woman in her fifties, who must have recently arrived to Nihue Rao, enters the dining hall, orders a plate of breakfast and sits down at the next table.

"With my heart cleared, a second phase to the ceremony commenced. During this time, I really had my ass handed to me," Guy says. "I felt a lot of shame as I was being told I needed to overcome my selfish reasons for coming down here. I heard the plant say, 'So asshole, you thought you'd come down here and drink this brew, and then go home and brag to your friends about it? You thought you'd become the *cool guy* to all your New Age friends, asshole?' As I was being delivered these tough messages, I became increasingly embarrassed, so much so that I went back to my room to change out of the ceremonial costume. I didn't feel worthy of wearing the Shipibo clothing. I was a fraud."

"After I changed and purged, Ana appeared at my door and brought me back to the maloca for my song. I felt a great sense of humility," Guy explains and his voice quivers; my own eyes now full with tears. "I thought the medicine was wearing off, but I now realize that the first two parts of the ceremony were prefaces to this third part. Mother Ayahuasca needed to know that I was open and humble before she'd let me see what she was about to show me. She needed to know that I wouldn't take the visions only to feed my own narcissistic ego."

"The geometric patterns from my first ceremony returned and I was being instructed to look more closely at what was happening. I was asked, 'What are you looking at?' And then, I realized that I was looking at the Creator and how she brings forth life into this world. These geometric patterns were the building blocks for the universe itself. I watched her manufacture jaguars, trees, insects, fish, animals, plants, objects of all sorts, and eventually, people. I was experiencing God unmediated and I began to sob at the realization of what I was seeing." Guy pauses again to regain his composure.

"As the ceremony was coming to an end, I had one last revelation: I recognized that the designs I had been seeing, which were all incredibly laser-like and brilliant in color, were being seen through the eyes of a snake, that I was seeing them in a kind of ultraviolet light that snakes see. I had the strong feeling that the snake I was viewing things through was an anaconda. I was left with a feeling of mystery about what that meant. 'Am I an anaconda? Am I strangling the life and love out of certain people and relationships in my life?' I was left to wonder."

"You know," the newly arrived woman chimes in, "snakes and anacondas aren't necessarily evil creatures. They play an important role on our planet." She smiles at us and adds, "My name's Ceta."

As Guy and Ceta continue talking, I sit at the dining room table. Maritza, a female parrot, hops onto my extended index finger. For twenty-five minutes, she and I stare into each other's eyes, into each other's souls, and into the universe, the multiverse and everything as a whole. I pull her closer to better see her pupils expand and contract, and her red, blue, yellow, green, and white feathers so beautiful to behold. I love her and all things so deeply that I cry soft tears from the inside out. She knows just as well as I that we are all everything and interconnected and that any separation between us is merely an illusion.

"That's amazing, Mike," Tatyana says, as she points to Maritza perched on my finger. "Normally, she doesn't like men."

Sleep-deprived, but energetic, I stroll around the sunny grounds of Nihue Rao. Around the outside of the building that houses the lounge and some offices, I come across Ersilia and an array of jewelry, garments, and tapestries. With a beaming smile, Ersilia hugs me and points to the jewelry, and then herself while speaking Spanish. Her words mean little to me, but I gather that all of the beautiful items on display are her creations. I peruse the jewelry in search of gifts for Linnea. All of it is intricate and beautiful, but I struggle to find something suitable. Ersilia pulls out a black and red beaded necklace with a small black heart hanging from the beads.

Perfect… I smile and nod.

I continue to look, but am unable to find anything that speaks to me. Ersilia pulls out one bracelet, and then another, both of which I know Linnea will love. I give Ersilia a thumbs up and the shaman sets the bracelets next to the necklace.

Now that I have some gifts for my love, I browse for something for myself. Ersilia pulls out a necklace with differently-shaped beige, black, and red beads and an animal's tooth for an ornament.

"Si," I say, unsure how the shaman knew I had started looking for a piece for myself.

Ersilia signals with her hands the number seventy and I give her eighty American dollars for the four pieces of jewelry. She embraces me once more and kisses my forehead.

Strolling the grounds, the hot sun warms my skin, and I feel a deep and powerful connection with the celestial ball of fire. I look at the towering trees and witness their efforts in extending upwards and closer to the energy source, everything more alive than a few days prior. A dog runs past me and barks "hello" as I contemplate the structural similarities between our solar system and the atoms that comprise it. Our sun, with its orbiting planets, nearly identical in design to a nucleus and its orbiting electrons. *The microcosm is the macrocosm*, I think, a phrase I've been saying since I was seventeen.

I think about the uncanny structural resemblance between our brains' neural networks and the organization of galaxies and stars. I consider how our highways connecting cities function similarly to arteries and veins connecting organs. I daydream of asteroids colliding with and fertilizing planets with DNA and life the same way a sperm cell fertilizes an ovarian egg[15]. Joyful tears swell in my eyes as I feel grateful for the repeating nature of nature itself, its obviously intelligent design, and my place in all of it.

---

15   It's largely speculated that DNA did not originate on Planet Earth, but instead arrived here via asteroid 3.5 billion years ago. With their tails, asteroids bear a striking resemblance to sperm cells.

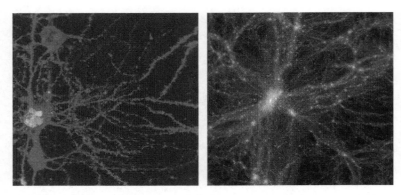

(Left) The neural networks of a mouse's brain.

(Right) Snapshot of the universe. The dots are galaxy clusters while the surrounding web is comprised of thousands of stars, galaxies and dark matter.

I think back to the trees and feel grateful for the oxygen they supply me with and I consider the diverse Amazonian ecosystem that is home to Mother Ayahuasca, the vessel to new understandings that I am so thankful to have met. I now realize what my intention for our third Ayahuasca ceremony will be. I intend to show gratitude for all things: Mother Ayahuasca, the shamans, our group, the universe, and the creator.

At 4:00 pm, I go for my pre-ceremony flower bath. The cool water refreshes my skin while the aromatic petals tickle my nostrils. Serenity overcomes me and I am ready to nap. Walking in the direction of my bed, Rafa informs me that Ricardo has just returned from Iquitos and that we're going to have conversacion— six hours later than scheduled.

With everyone gathered inside the maloca, Ricardo apologizes for being late. He was delayed by a rainstorm and washed out roads. Sitting near Ricardo, Ceta introduces herself to our group. She is a shaman who works in South and North America. She has been involved with Ayahuasca since the 1990s and has worked with the likes of Terence McKenna, amongst other seekers and psychonauts.

Rafa opens the conversacion by saying, "Since we're starting late, we'll try to keep things short."

He smiles and then invites me to start.

I quickly summarize my experience before Rafa translates it into Spanish. Ricardo looks at me with a smile.

Jon moves past the foot of his mattress to sit on the hard floor before he shares his experience.

"My intention going into the ceremony was karmic cleansing and emotional cleansing. I threw up about ten minutes into the ceremony. Immediately after that, I started to experience a lot of heavy, dense energy, a lot of fear, a lot of doubt. And I was pretty much in a place of darkness until I came up for my song. As soon as the shamans started singing to me, I went into another purge and started to vomit and throw up into my bucket—all of that negative energy and fear I was having previously. The rest of the night involved me continuing the whole healing process." Jon moves his hands in a rotating manner. "My intention for tonight is to strengthen the connection with my higher self and to gain more clarity on my purpose."

After Jon, Tatyana, accompanied by her journal, is next in the rotation.

"What I went through can only be compared to Hell," she starts, her voice calm and collected. "Waves of panic and fear overcame me, a suffering beyond anything I thought possible. I prayed for help from everyone I could: Archangel Michael, Gabriel, my spiritual guide, God. I struggled to remember and articulate their names, as if some force was trying to prevent me from any contact with those who could help. I kept praying. I prayed as best as I could, calling out their names, I repeated, 'God, God, God, God, God.' I couldn't believe that this was happening to me." As Tatyana shares, I observe a shift in my thinking: normally, biblical references to God turn me off, but as my friend relates her story, I'm empathetic to her beliefs. I don't identify with the beliefs, but I respect where Tatyana comes from.

She continues, "I felt like something was trying to steal my soul. I've never felt anything like this before. I resisted believing that this was happening to me. I was waiting for somebody from the maloca to help me. I really needed help, but for some reason, couldn't ask for it. I thought that every person in the maloca must've known what I was going through, but I was completely alone. And now I understand why. It was a lesson of independence. I overcame a real challenge by myself. Last night, Mother Ayahuasca taught me how to truly appreciate life, to be happy about being in my own body, about the fact that my mind is bright and my soul is with me."

"The feeling of true bliss that I'm experiencing can't be compared to anything else," Tatyana continues, sitting cross-legged with a straight spine. "So much warmth, love, and lessons, as if a mother intentionally threw her child into a tornado of vanity for its own benefit. And when everything was finally over and the lesson was learned, she, witnessing the suffering of her baby, surrounded it with the deepest tenderness. I am grateful for life; grateful for every single day, every single second, every in-breath and out-breath."

Tatyana flips the page in her journal, and then speaks further. "I was able to clear a rooted fear. I wrapped the situation from my youth when I was almost raped and killed into a green grid and sent it to God. Earlier, Ricardo taught us to wrap negative energies in green nets or grids and send them away. It really works. I released that fear."

"When my time came for an icaro, I wanted Ricardo to sing it to me, nobody else but him. And he did. I sat across from him, lotus position, and noticed the silence around me. It felt like a blessing for what I had to go through. As though all the shamans knew about what happened to me and looked at me as though I was a warrior who became a thousand times stronger in a moment. Ricardo began to sing and I felt a rainbow around me and a crystal within, which became clearer and more diamond-like through the survived experience."

"And if you'll allow me, just a few more things." Tatyana looks to Rafa who nods.

"I learned that a true healer's heart is soft. The true healer lets the person heal himself. I learned that I am a child of God, playing the game called life. Our world is a playground and everything we wish for comes true. Abundance of love, satisfaction, happiness, peace, wealth and health is inherited by us since we came to Earth. There is absolutely nothing to be afraid of."

After Rafa translates Tatyana's experience to Ricardo, Ricardo smiles and nods to Tatyana and she laughs.

Then, Dan starts with his experience.

"After having cleared some negative energies during the New Year's Eve ceremony, last night was about opening my path and inviting creativity so that I can find a way to make this project successful enough to take care of us. I feel like I'm on the right path, so my intention for tonight will be similar to last night's."

Continuing in the circle, Sid explains the purging, and the physical and psychological breakdown he endured before his eyes light up and his voice quickens.

"The interesting thing about it, which I'm just realizing right now, is that my intention going into the night was to cultivate the observer in myself. Although I was in this extremely difficult place mentally—I kept repeating to myself, 'I'm losing my sanity; I don't know what's real; I don't know what's not,'—it's almost like the observer in me talked me through it. This observer, combined with the icaros, and the fact that I knew I had my friends and family around me, allowed me to navigate through the insanity and through the emotions that I was feeling; which is so profound because…" Sid shifts on his mattress. "I didn't even realize that until just now…" He straightens his spine. "And that was exactly what my intention was." Sid pauses and takes a big breath. "So, I feel gratitude for the shamans, and I feel a very strong connection with my friends and the bonds I've made here."

Following the translations, Carl shares his experience.

"Visions, white lights, yellow lights, and for the first time, I actually saw some shapes. I saw a lot of rows of eyes, like tons and tons of rows of eyes. I saw rows of skulls. After that, I thought everything was done; I felt completely level. About two hours later, I was hit much more intensely by the Ayahuasca. I was a little overwhelmed, a little confused, dizzy, disoriented for another half hour or an hour—that hit me pretty hard. Eventually, that faded. That was the experience. Tonight, my focus is to be very open minded and to continue the cleanse."

After Carl, Guy shares the experience I heard him recount earlier in the dining hall and expresses a sincere thanks to the shamans for having helped him clear the blockages around his heart. Ricardo responds, and through Rafa's translation, thanks Guy for staying awake through the cleansing process.

"You showed strength and a willingness to improve, which made our work possible," Ricardo says through Rafa's voice.

I realize that my previous assumption of Guy being self-absorbed to think Ricardo's vomit was about him was unfounded.

Guy then explains his intention for our third and final ceremony.

"This evening, I want to learn how to take all of this and integrate it into my life and how to be of service to my community. I want to take these insights and put them into action for the betterment of myself, my community, and perhaps the global community."

Ricardo nods to Guy before addressing everyone in the maloca. After the shaman finishes, Rafa translates the words to English: "We've had quite the journey thus far. I really like this group. You're all synchronized. Last night, most of you had trying times. Some difficult situations, and yet you all sit here with smiling faces and willing to share. You haven't been here very long, but we've covered a lot of ground, and tonight represents your last ceremony before you leave. We will work to integrate the experiences you've had so far, so that when you leave this place, you will do so with grace and purpose. Again, pay attention. Work with the icaros, your intentions, and focus on your journey."

As conversacion concludes, my eyelids feel like they're full of lead and I find a hammock outside the maloca to rest in.

Seemingly no time later, I wake to a night sky, crisp air, and the realization that our final ceremony draws near. I change into my ceremonial pants, grab four mapachos, and the necklace I purchased for Linnea earlier in the day.

I enter the maloca and take my place on my mattress. I look around at the familiar faces inside our sacred space, and I see a new girl, named Hilary, who arrived earlier this afternoon. Jon and I exchange excited, joyous laughter, and I feel peaceful.

I intend to show gratitude for all things: Mother Ayahuasca, the shamans, our group, the universe, the creator. I intend to clear my darkness and open up my path.

Erjomenes pours what I know is the right amount of Ayahuasca into the glass, blows his intent into the brew, and hands me the drink. I whisper my intent and welcome the mother of the rainforest into my body, into my soul.

On my mattress, I sit with legs extended and my back against the pillows. Jon walks toward the maloca's center.

I intend to show gratitude for all things: Mother Ayahuasca, the shamans, our group, the universe, the creator. I intend to clear my darkness and open up my path. Have a wonderful journey, Jon. Thank you.

I bring my hands to prayer pose and feel a deep gratitude for all things.

I repeat my mantra and thanks as Tatyana, Dan, Sid, Carl, Guy, Hilary, Ceta, Ana, Erjomenes, Ersilia, Ricardo, and Rafa walk to the room's center to have their brew.

I set my intention once more: *I intend to show gratitude for all things: Mother Ayahuasca, the shamans, our group, the universe, the creator. I intend to clear my darkness and open up my path. Thank you. I am ready, Mother Ayahuasca. Welcome.*

In a meditative pose with eyes closed, my mind and body are still. I am supremely light. After thirty minutes, I lie down and the icaros begin. I chuckle softly and hum along, the tune and tone coming through me.

I see the back of a giant white bird with brown spots staring through the open screened door of a big wooden doorframe. The doorframe is part of a house built for a giant and the bird is more vivid than life has ever been. So vivid and so real that the vision frightens me for a moment. The bird disappears as soft, peaceful colors fill my mind. A bright white panda comes into view, startlingly vivid, against a bright green backdrop. A second panda sits on top of the first's shoulders. It's a cute and funny image, but for some reason, a bit scary. And then I learn why: a third giant panda appears on top of the second's shoulders with dark brown fur and thick black rims around his eyes, unquestionably evil. I wrap the image in a green net, uprooting the pandas and sending them away.

Peacefully, I lie for an hour or more. I feel boundless gratitude for everything. I listen to the shamans belt out Ayahuasca's songs, immersed in the moment. I feel only peace and see soft colors. I realize that though this experience doesn't seem particularly profound, I'd be content if this were the extent of the trip.

What else could I want?

Ana approaches to invite me for my song. She tells me to bring my bucket, though I suspect I won't need it. I stand, and for the first time during ceremony, navigating the physical world is unchallenging. I sit cross-legged in front of Ricardo, his physical energy and a subtle spirit energy apparent. He sings and I express gratitude. I sway softly with the music, a smile on my face. The peaceful song and dance last about six minutes before I walk back to my mattress and thank Ana for her assistance. Lying back down, I'm confident that Ricardo's song will elicit some lingering effects. *I think he's showing me something.* I see a variety of energies, some bright, some dark and scary looking. I net the scary ones away. Time moves, the number of scary spirits dwindles and my gratitude magnifies. I feel my body as the membrane it is and become permeable.

Carl vomits five times. *Be well, my friend.*

I'm physically and mentally open and I feel energy pass through me.

I sit up to watch Guy struggle as he stands from his mattress and stumbles his first couple of steps. As he staggers toward the door, a shadow stands from the mattress and strides toward Guy from behind. The shadow walks inside Guy's body and merges with the physical form; Guy instantly regains his coordination, and then walks sure-footed to the washroom.

Wow.

I hear Jon crying as the right side of my cranium becomes completely permeable. A liquid-like portal opens from my head and forms a direct connection to Jon. His sobs now seem more potent, so I think comforting thoughts for my suffering compadre. Jon's tears and energy intensify and nearly overwhelm me. Knowing I need to protect myself from absorbing his pain, I work to close the portal. I rub my hand on my head, and though the volume of his sobs dampens, the connection persists.

I focus my attention on the spirits in my field. A giant orange-with-a-hint-of-yellow arachnoid creature floats above me. I can't decide whether he's good or bad. Despite my uncertainty, I don't stop the spider as he approaches my abdomen and crosses the permeable barrier into my stomach. It seems like the spider is working on something inside me, and I wonder whether Ricardo performs some kind of cleanse, something to help me out.

A dark-blue-with-a-hint-of-purple spider floats in to the right of the orange one, and I'm similarly uncertain of this new creature's energy. I'm less comfortable. *Am I too permeable? Too accepting?* Disappearing from my visual field, the spiders rush into my right hip and my hip starts to ache. I move around trying to rid the pain in the physical realm, but it's not working. I'm not panicked, but I am concerned. The ache is quite strong. I consider asking Rafa for help.

What if I've let something in? Something that I don't know how to get rid of?

Not wanting to disturb Rafa, I lie and think. I try to remove the spiders by visualizing a green net to wrap them in. I pull at the spiders a few times but they barely budge. I focus on positive spirits in the vicinity, but they're merely a distraction. This pain won't alleviate itself and it's aching badly, deep in my bones. Unsure what to do, I wonder about the safety of becoming conscious of the universe in this way.

Is this even real? I'm on Ayahuasca. Does this spirit world actually exist?

Sober and crystal-clear headed, I know the answer is yes.

Is it safe to be here? Should I have opened Pandora's Box? Have I made a wrong decision?

But because this realm exists, I cannot regret having entered this space. Ignorance is *not* bliss, and as a forever explorer, I crave the truth. I want to see more, understand more, feel more, and know more. I cannot pretend there isn't something profound here. I'm incapable of settling and have no desire to do so anyways. This ache though, this infiltration: I need to exorcize it. I consider Rafa's help once more, but I sense it will be best to solve the problem on my own.

Dan stumbles from his mattress toward the center of the maloca. He takes two steps forward, stumbles one back and another to the side. A shadow stands from the mattress behind him, strides toward him and merges with the physical form, and Dan's confident stride is instantly regained.

Jon starts laughing a strange laugh. I squirm both due to my hip ache and the gross warmth of my neighbor's noises. Jon's laugh feels like a large, evil and hairy place, and I feel like I'm inside it. He seems possessed and I want to escape. His being gay comes to mind as I become increasingly uncomfortable—not because I'm homophobic, but because I feel uncomfortably close, like an unwanted force has invaded my personal boundaries. Two emotionless tears fall from my eyes.

I sit up, move to the foot of my mattress and twist my body to the left and into a partial ball, trying to separate myself from Jon's laughter. Despite the increased distance, the connection remains as intense, my efforts in the physical realm bearing seemingly no consequence.

Should I ask the shamans to request that Jon be quiet?

I'm sure everyone in the room is cognizant of Jon's bellows, though I doubt anyone else is as intimately engaged and disturbed. I think about asking Jon to stop laughing his possessed and evil laugh, but I can't bring myself to interfere with his journey. I twinge, bob, and rub my head. I know that I'm physically behaving like a tormented person, like someone in a white-padded room. But, my mind is clear. I know this will pass.

From across the maloca, an energy moves in our direction. Ceta kneels down and asks if she can chant to Jon. Jon gives a polite "no, thank you," and I hang my head. I had anticipated his acceptance and my own relief. Ceta lingers before standing and I roll onto my left side, questioning my friend's decision. I watch Ceta walk away and see swirling serpents surrounding her. I sense she shares an intimate relationship with snakes.

Jon resumes laughing and I remain uncomfortable. His laugh is so strange.

Wait, why am I so bothered by his laughter and the experience he's having?
Is it really Jon's problem that I'm disturbed, or is it my own?

A green net yanks the spiders from my hip and the pain dissipates! Jon's laugh no longer bothers me as I move outside of it! Everything, every and all things, become maximally peaceful! Lying down, I jolt that falling jolt that occurs the moment before sleep. But, I'm not sleepy, and instead of falling, it feels like I'm rising. I jolt again and again and see flashes of lightning. I'm so at peace and I feel so light, like gravity has released its grip from me. I jolt seven more times to more flashes of lightning before I sit up cross-legged near the foot of my bed, wide-awake and full of bliss. I'm decidedly in the maloca with complete control of my physical body and aware of everyone else in the room. I'm also decidedly in another realm—a realm that fills the inside of the maloca like a palpable clear film overlaying the physical structure. A new realm of blissfully comforting familiarity. This new realm, undeniably infinite, breathes the most soothing cadence.

The icaros silence. Everything is at peace as crickets chirp in this heavenly space. Strangely shaped organisms are scattered throughout. Depictions of these organisms can be found on much of the Shipibo art throughout Nihue Rao and Iquitos, the art that until now had no meaning for me. Each one of the organisms breathes and each one has a warm soul so welcoming—an invitation that can only be described as nirvana. Feeling any more at home, I know, is impossible. I don't remember ever having seen this place before, but I'm supremely familiar with it. I've never liked the following words due to their religious connotations, but I am in *heaven*. I see and I'm with *God*. I am at the Source. I *know* this to be true. I do not think, believe, hope or wonder; I *know* it's true—a knowing that far exceeds any knowledge I've ever held—my understanding of knowledge redefined.

Jon giggles and says, "Si. Si. Yes!" as his soul smiles with radiant white light and mine does too. I've ascended, transcended to a place in the stars, and I know that everything Jon has hinted at is true.

"Yes! Haha. Yes!" Jon says aloud. I can tell he's receiving affirmation of everything he's ever thought and known. He sits up and I see his body's silhouette with sharp clarity. We are floating amongst the stars in a cosmic indigo aura. I stare at Jon as we communicate telepathically and share our gratitude for God and for our Higher Selves, another term I've never used before[16].

Looking upward, I know the meaning of life and I realize every decision I've made has been the right one. Every decision I've ever made has led to this moment. My whole life has been a quest to *now* and my physical world's mind has constantly communicated with my Higher Self without my conscious awareness. All the existential contemplations I've had, which account for about half of my waking hours on this Earth, are answered.

All of those contemplations were my physical mind receiving communication from my Higher Self, my Higher Self guiding my physical self to this moment. Every time I looked up at the stars as a child at our Parry Sound cottage; when I laid in the hammock of my parents' backyard under a starry night sky; when I stood ankle deep in the Atlantic Ocean off Daytona Beach on my eighteenth birthday with my head in the clouds and feet in the sand; when I swam around the crystal clear water of Halong Bay, Vietnam alone and under a full moon at 4:00 am; and when I star gazed from the dock in Huntsville. Every time I had that deep knowing that I will be all right and that we are forever; every day at Burning Man when I reveled in the divine interconnectedness of all things—Jon shouts, "Yes! Si!"—every second I spend with

---

16   I recognize that God is a charged word. For the record, my experience has nothing to do with the religious associations of the concept. While many religions offer some beautiful teachings, I do not identify with any of the institutions. My experience continues to be a spiritual one, not a religious one.

Linnea; every time I've been compelled to dance, to express myself and to write and share my story, my Higher Self was guiding me. My Higher Self is guiding me to now.

I know the meaning of life.

Jon shouts in a whisper, "Yes!"

Ecstatic tears come over me as I fall back onto my pillow and my soul screams: *THANK YOU!*

I cry fearlessly, for fear has been abolished. There's no such thing as fear, not even the potential for it. My whole life up until now has been one of effort. Now, I can simply *be*. The minds of my physical and Higher Selves have reunited and ascended to the heavens. I realize what Jon said about the final ascension of soul into star is true.

Jon shouts, "Yes! Si!"

I recognize that everything is belief and everything is easy. Anything and everything is accomplished by believing so strongly that one *knows* it to be true. Just like when I was first learning handstands, I couldn't handstand until I believed I could. And, I couldn't believe I could handstand until I believed I was qualified. As I practiced each day, my belief in my qualification increased until one day, I believed so strongly in my qualification that I believed I could handstand, and all doubt was eliminated. My belief was so strong that I *knew* I could handstand. With every fiber of my being, I knew I could, and thus I was able to.

And thus, I can only *know* what is real. And now I know I can ascend to the stars. I have transcended my body and the physical space.

But what do I do once I become a star?

I realize I've been a star for the last twenty seconds of physical Earth time and I return to the heaven dimension I was in before.

Ah, I don't get to know that yet because I'm not ready to leave the physical world.

I recognize the importance of detachment from all things and from all people. This is not to say that I can't connect with people or have meaningful relationships, but that I need not depend on them. All I need is myself, my Higher Self.

This realization shows me this journey has evolved past a personal one. My mission is to share my story and to help others realize their Higher Selves.

In simple terms, I want to help people connect with themselves. I have to execute this mission with the utmost love, compassion, and patience: not everyone is ready for this kind of information. I'm aware that these ideas and this knowledge could be perceived as insane. With those who are resistant, I must display even greater love, compassion, and patience. My path does not involve indoctrination; my path simply involves helping those who are ready to be shown. These ideas are foreign to most people's understanding of reality, and thus, I will practice care with the way I communicate. I am not worried. I am so happy.

Thank you... Thank you. My intention for gratitude tonight was also a message from my Higher Self.

I sit up again with a beaming smile. Looking around the room, I see everything so clearly inside night's lack of light. Guy gets up again, and is again uncoordinated. He wobbles three steps before his black shadow gets up from the mattress and re-connects with his physical form, and once again, Guy regains his sober step. The display reminds me of Peter Pan and his shadow.

Love pours outward from me to all things.

I recognize how incredibly deep telepathy is. We are all always communicating all the time. When one thinks something, that energy travels through the universe. Thoughts become things, just like every structure I've ever stood in originated as a thought. Everything originated as a thought. While we're not consciously aware of all the thoughts our friends and family think, our subconscious and unconscious pick them up, and eventually they manifest in the conscious mind one way or another.

I've been communicating telepathically with Jon and the shamans for the past ninety minutes.

I send Carl a thought: *Hey man, can you hear me?* Instantly, I hear Carl's voice: *"Yea man."* Holy shit! Whoa. *Ok, if you can hear me, stand up and walk over to me.* Carl does not stand. I realize I'm not communicating with his conscious mind, but somewhere in his sub or unconscious. The thought has been sent and somewhere inside his mind has received it. I suspect he'll come eventually.

I recognize that ideas take time to manifest themselves in physical reality—for we humans typically operate in the third dimension. Just like it took time for me to train my body to handstand—to make it believe that I can handstand—it takes time and a process to transform the idea of a skyscraper into a physical one. And, it will take time for my telepathic request for Carl to walk over to act on his physical body.

I consider veganism. For the first time, I accept veganism as a potentially healthy way of life. The argument against veganism regarding lack of B vitamins and amino acids simply operates in a paradigm that operates independently of reality. If one has the proper beliefs, one does not need the B vitamins or amino acids supplied by meat. Most people just think they do. N always equals 1.[17]

Eating meat is unnecessary. But, is it wrong? If killing a plant for food is permissible, why would killing an animal not be the same?

An answer swells: *All plants form one consciousness, and thus, they offer themselves to us. When a plant is consumed, the overall consciousness remains, and only physical and inconsequential matter is lost. When an animal is killed, an entire consciousness dies. Thus every time I eat an animal, I eat death.*

---

17   N=1 means that if a scientific theory shows that an input yields the same output ninety-nine times in a row, this does not guarantee that the one-hundredth sample will yield the same; i.e. every situation is unique.

I ask: *But, if everything originates from God, then am I not eating God each time I nourish myself with animal or plant? If so, then how could it be wrong to eat animal?*

The response I receive is: *It is not necessarily wrong, but the animal does not want to die. So, by eating animal, I darken my spirit and hinder my evolution toward ascension and the post-physical.*

I resist this notion, partly because I'm still attached to my body, and partly because my current diet allowed me to ascend to this point, and I know if I had chosen to, I could have remained an ascended star. Plus, I received confirmation during my first ceremony that my digestive tract is on point and that I've been making my body a welcoming place for light spirits. Because I'm an athlete, I think that animal consumption improves my health, and I know a healthy body and mind are essential to ascension. *But, maybe one day, I'll switch to veganism.* I ponder fearlessly.

The shamans begin to sing again. I am so grateful to have had their guidance throughout my time in Nihue Rao. My journey wouldn't have been possible without them. Their icaros and their presence help shape the realms I've gained access to, like a spaceship allowing me to explore beyond Earth's atmosphere. As I listen to their song, my mind and body remain in heaven. I laugh with Jon.

The ceremony ends and Ricardo lights a candle. Carl walks over and sits down to speak with me. He received my earlier telepathic thought. We talk in a place of joy and I'm still in heaven. My Higher Self now consciously guides me. There's no such thing as doubt. When something makes me feel good, I'm doing the right thing. When I'm uncomfortable or sad, I need to get back on course.

Jon sleeps while others in the maloca sing heavenly songs. Hilary, in particular, soothes our souls with a voice from above before Carl sings to Rafa's guitar playing.

After everyone falls asleep, I put in my earbuds and am guided to play Wintersleep's "Weighty Ghost." I'm filled with joy and covered in goose bumps as I listen to the song, and realize that my falling in love with it seven years ago was another means by which my Higher Self communicated with me. I play *Anjunadeep Volume 5* and realize that my favorite music has always been a means by which my Higher Self communicates. I scroll through the album titles beneath *Anjunadeep Volume 5*. In consecutive order on my iPod: *The Art of Storytelling, Art of Storytelling, The Art of Storytelling, Art of Storytelling* (yes, it's there four times), *Art Official Intelligence, Ascension, Ascension (Side C)*—holy shit, tears swell at the obviousness of coincidence not existing—*At the Speed of Life, Atlantis, ATLiens, Audioslave, August and Everything After* (referring to my spiritual growth catalyzed by Burning Man), *Away from the Sun, B Day, Back to Bedlam.*

I recognize that any skeptic would view this list as coincidental and think that I'm imposing meaning, but the skeptic's view and my knowledge differ in wavelength.

I lie back and let the music fill my soul as I drift to sleep.

JANUARY 4, 2014

I wake at 6:00 am to dance around the maloca while listening to Sasha's *Invol<3r* album as the sky pours rain outside. I flow with the rhythm of the music, the rhythm of my body, and the rhythm of the universe, spinning, twirling, stepping, leaping, handstanding, somersaulting, waving, jumping, and gliding.

Later in the morning, we have conversacion.

Guy begins the sharing.

"Last night's ceremony was a logical progression from the first and second one—like act one, act two, and now act three of some cosmic play. I got a lot of visuals, scenarios, and teachings based on my intention of learning how to integrate what I've experienced into my life when I get back home. I was taught some important lessons about the mother and the sense of loss she experiences when she has to let her offspring go out into the world. Toward the end of the evening, I had a very dark experience that involved some tarantulas and spiders and the feeling that I had been poisoned. I don't know if those spiders represented something inside me or not."

Rafa translates Guy's experience to Ricardo, and then Ricardo's response back to Guy and the group. "Those spiders were not something inside of you. They were a dark energy from outside the space that infiltrated the maloca. We worked to dispel those. A couple of years ago, those spiders invaded the maloca regularly. That's why we installed those webs up there." Rafa points to the structures in the ceiling that I thought looked like ten-spoke wagon wheels. "Every once in a while, the spiders come back. This is one reason why awareness is important: to protect oneself from dark energies."

Carl speaks next.

"Last night was good. Initially, it was pretty smooth sailing and I made it my mission to try and stay level the entire time, which didn't really work out." He laughs. "After about two hours, I had a pretty aggressive purge—first time I've puked in five years, actually. I tried to fight it. I did not want to succumb to the medicine, but the Ayahuasca overpowered me and made me throw up. It felt good though, like a deep cleanse. My body feels cleaner than it's ever been," Carl says with deep satisfaction in his voice and eyes.

Sid shares next.

"Overall, it was a pretty positive experience. Physically, it was similar to my second ceremony. I experienced some vomiting, some sweating, and some diarrhea, which lasted for about half an hour. After that, I felt leveled out and I took a second dose—as advised by Ana—to open up my vision, since I had already experienced the physical purge. Then, I started seeing some things. Jon started laughing and giggling in this weird, almost possessed state, and I envisioned him as this phoenix who was breaking out of his shell and burning upwards; there was a lot of energy coming from Jon during the ceremony." Sid looks to Jon.

"Wow, my friends call me a phoenix," Jon says, smiling, as Sid continues. "Then, I experienced a moment of extreme gratitude, particularly for Carl and Mike. I remember telling Carl that I was very grateful to have him here. And then, I experienced a period of extreme awareness: I woke up and rose from my seat, and I was breathing very heavily, very calm and gazing around the room. I was almost in a trance state with the icaros coming from Erjomenes. Overall, it was an incredible experience, the most peace I've felt. I was exhausted, so I fell asleep for a while. At the end of the ceremony, we just hung out, played some guitar, and it was really relaxing."

Dan explains that his experience was a continuation of the previous ceremony. "I'm just focused on making this project work, and figuring out how to best help people."

"Last night was a peaceful experience with some softer insights," Tatyana articulates, having had a much milder ceremony compared to her previous one.

Jon sits up to talk about his ceremony.

"My third and final ceremony was amazing. It was pure; it was bliss. I received everything I had asked for with my intent. Everything was fulfilled. I pretty much had a reawakening: a major, major, major breakthrough." He smiles from ear to ear. "The laughing y'all heard was me laughing at myself. I was laughing at myself because I realized my fears and my doubts, and I realized that they were no longer needed."

After I share the journey and revelations of my third ceremony, and mention that I also encountered the spiders, Ricardo expresses delight for all the experiences shared by our group. With every Ayahuasca experience, the individual can grow, regardless of whether or not the teachings are apparent. The medicine alone is not the answer, but the teachings we must now carry forward will help us become our true selves.

As Ricardo speaks, I feel what he says, despite my inability to speak Spanish.

Most of the group has left the maloca, but Jon and I remain to talk about our experiences.

"Jon, first off, we were having a telepathic conversation for over an hour last night, right?" I ask, wanting to confirm his mind was as conscious of the experience as mine was.

"Of course!" He laughs. "That was incredible!"

"There were no boundaries between our minds. I could see, feel and sense everything inside your mind. I had access to all of your thoughts. And, I know you had access to all of mine. Our consciousness is not restricted to our brains. Our consciousness resides beyond our bodies."

"Si, brother. Consciousness is co-created."

As we continue our conversation, every word Jon speaks fills me with joy. I empathize so deeply that it feels like I'm the one speaking his words. Whenever I talk, Jon's eyes light up and he laughs.

"It's like fear has been abolished."

"Even the potential for fear no longer exists."

"Every decision throughout my entire life has been the right one, the necessary one."

"The alternatives weren't even possible."

"I know the meaning of life."

"And I've been to heaven."

"Thank you for being such a great teacher."

Jon is one of the best teachers I've encountered. The patience with which he communicates allowed me to remain open-minded enough to hear him out. Not once did I feel like he was trying to persuade me to his way of thinking. Throughout our time in Peru, he simply shared in hopes of helping. The man's throat chakra beams light. I recognize that mine does, too.

Storytelling is my path.

"Tatyana, do you think there are any children nearby that would enjoy some bouncy balls?" I ask.

"Ricardo's children are right over there," she says and points behind the dining hall. "I'm sure they'd love some."

I approach the young girl and boy, both of whom giggle and bounce around. I say "Hola" and hand them each two balls.

"Gracias," says the girl.

"Gracias," says the boy.

"Gracias," I say. We all smile as I walk away.

The moto-taxi ride back to Iquitos is tumultuous, a rainstorm having flooded much of the road a couple of hours before. Our vehicle jolts and jostles, mud flies in all directions, and we get stuck a few times before local children help push us along.

"I'm on edge, Sandman." Sid says, as his heart races during our bumpy ride. I turn around to see Jon smiling and laughing in the moto-taxi behind us. I smile and laugh too, knowing there's nothing to worry about.

I contemplate surrender: everything feels much easier, much simpler now that I've surrendered to the universe, the moment, and myself.

I think about déjà vu, of which I've had a few during my time in Peru. Deep down, I think everyone knows, or at least senses, that the familiarity of déjà vu is not coincidental. It is not something to be dismissed, for déjà vu is not inconsequential. I've long questioned time's linearity and I'm beginning to think that déjà vus are messages from my Higher Self to show me that I'm on the right path.

Back in Iquitos for our last supper as a group, the city celebrates its 150th year and the energy is intense. Never have I felt so permeable, and I think Tatyana, Jon, Carl, and Sid feel similarly. Dealing with all the world's various energies requires patience and I already feel myself being tested. I've only slept for three and a half hours in the past fifty-eight, so I suspect my lack of rest contributes to the challenge.

I watch Guy sip a beer, and I'm somewhat bothered by his

choice to drink alcohol before quickly remembering that it's not my place to judge him.

After dinner, we take a few pictures and exchange "so longs" before Sid, Carl, and I hop in a car en route to the airport. I feel nostalgia for Peru and the friends I've met. In the back of the cab, Sid and Carl belt out improvised mock emo songs like "Trust Issues", "I Hate Everything", and "My Shoes are too Tight" as I sit in the front seat. Together, my two friends form the duo *Lack of Motivation*, guaranteed to be a YouTube sensation.

While we sing and laugh, a dog runs in front of our car. Our driver tries to avoid the collision, but we smash into and drive over the animal. I feel the animal roll against the car floor beneath my feet, undoubtedly dead. Sadness passes through me as I appreciate the temporality of this physical realm. In this moment, and with heightened sensitivity, the death almost overwhelms me, but I know I'll be all right.

EPILOGUE

Shortly after returning to Toronto, I met with Charlie to discuss *I Wager That*. He was excited to hear about my experience, so I read him my journal. When I arrived at the vision of the porcelain man bursting through the swamp and shedding skin, I prefaced what came next by saying, "This might be difficult for you to hear." I recounted the part about my inadequate passion for making *IWT* a success and read the line, "And so, an open and honest conversation with Charlie needs to be had," with the intent of closing my journal to talk.

"Go on. We can talk about that after. I want to hear about the rest of the ceremony first," Charlie said. I read the rest of my journal before we addressed *IWT*. Charlie, one of my best friends for the past seven years, was understanding and appreciative of my honesty. He's going to pursue *IWT*—which has since changed names and evolved into something more philanthropic and much greater—with the passion required, and I will remain an advisor to his company. I'm confident he will achieve his goals.

* * *

Prior to my conversation with Charlie, the first thing I did after landing was invite Linnea over. We hadn't seen each other since before Christmas. She brought me the most beautiful gift I've ever received—a painting she made for me. We spent the next three days in a blissful and loving state, and she explained how she had experienced magnificent white light and a uniting of our souls during her New Year's Day meditation. That weekend, we had dinner with her mom and other family members, which was equally wonderful.

The following week, I sensed some distance, and when I picked her up one night to go see a play called *This Is It*, she hopped in my car and delivered the news that she had had a conversation with a former lover. The lover, whom she had once considered spending her life with, had called to explain that he was ready to change. He was ready to be the man she had needed him to be before they parted ways some months prior.

I realized she was telling me this because she was thinking about giving him another chance. I sat silently as I wondered whether the Earth was flat, if my understanding of reality was being challenged as strongly as when I witnessed a new dimension full of infinite spirits for the first time!

Had I misinterpreted our connection? I must have. Walking away from what we shared was not only impossible in my mind, but even the contemplation of doing so was not something that existed.

I must have loved her more than she loved me. I thought this without believing it.

I know she felt what I felt. It's obvious.

After ten minutes in a state of shock, I found it in me to speak. Linnea and I skipped the play and spent the next four hours talking. She confirmed that I had not misinterpreted the love we shared and that this new development did not take away from the experience we had, but that she felt a compulsion to try things out with her former lover. She resolved that she would take some time to think before making a decision.

During the days we spent apart, I spent a lot of time meditating and going for walks. There were some tears and painful moments, but overall, I was clear-headed. I knew that whether or not Linnea and I stayed together, I would still be me and I would be all right. Though I wanted to be with her, I did not want that to be her reason for being with me. I did not want a relationship in which she wondered about being with her former lover. I read a quote from Free Spirit's *Keys to Immortality*—the book that Jon gifted me and that I read within days of returning to Toronto—which provided reassurance: "Love is to ultimately allow all beings to experience their own choices."

Driving to Linnea's the following Thursday, I wasn't sure what we would decide. I didn't know whether we could move forward as lovers after this time in question. When I arrived, she explained that her compulsion remained. We talked, expressed thanks, shed tears, and hugged for a couple of hours before I hopped in my car to go home. I released five powerful and painful sobs before calling my mom to chat about life's beauty.

Despite the loss of Linnea, I felt uplifted. I knew there would be pain, but I was unafraid of it. Wonderful lessons about detachment, impermanence, life, love, and myself would follow. I woke up the next morning with a smile on my face and the desire to dance. So, I danced for two hours around my living room.

I remain grateful for what Linnea and I shared. We both taught each other many wonderful things and I wish her the best moving forward.

* * *

In the summer of 2014, Jon moved to Hawaii where he continues with his spiritual ascension and working with crystal energies and jewelry.

* * *

In September 2014, Dan, Tatyana, and Pulse Tours officially opened their own Ayahuasca Adventure Center adjacent to the Peruvian Amazonian village of Libertad, which means "freedom" in Spanish. Appreciative of the work Pulse Tours does, Libertad's mayor gave Dan and his team a tract of waterfront land that offers beautiful open views, sunrises and sunsets over the river, easy boat access, close proximity to primary rainforest for jungle exploration and to the small villages of Libertad and Puerto Miguel for activities and cultural immersion. Pulse Tours employs local people, works with experienced shamans, is mindful of both the people and the environment, and provides a great boost to the local economy. Pulse Tours' guests continue to have life-changing experiences and the company is ranked highly on AyaAdvisor.org.

* * *

In October 2014, Guy officially moved on from his editor position at two environmental magazines in order to devote his time to writing about and pursuing his various interests, which include music, art, shamanism, and spirituality.

* * *

Sid, Carl, and I continue to grow as friends.

Sid's expanding his family business while also exploring the globe, other ventures, and connecting people in a way few people do. He and I again ventured to Burning Man in 2014, a magical and transformative experience that warrants a book of its own.

Carl works in sales and continues to produce music. He's dedicated to making cryptocurrency more accessible to the masses and is involved in *Vitaly*, a successful and growing jewelry and clothing company.

Carl and I recently became investors and the Vice Presidents of Sales and Marketing, respectively, for SunMoon Energy. We're a clean energy startup with the technologies, team, partnerships, and strategy to evolve energy and heal our planet. With our triple bottom line focus on people, planet, and profit, I believe we are one of the most exciting and necessary initiatives on the planet right now and feel blessed to be a part of it. My decision to focus on clean energy is largely informed by my experience and forever deepening connection with Ayahuasca.

* * *

I've been developing my spirituality through my daily meditation and movement practice, deepening my connection with the universe and my Higher Self. I've been forming close and loving relationships with an expanding number of wonderful people and am finding inspiration and peace in everyday life.

With each and every decision I make, I try to make the largest positive impact on the world that I can—being mindful of the fact that I need to take care of myself, be present, rest, and appreciate the journey.

My path remains one of storytelling and making human connection, of which this book is an integral part. I've also recently launched www.michaelsanders.co, an online resource filled with stories, meditations, dreams, and other content to help you find your enlightenment. I hope to connect with and help people around the world.

I hope to inspire you to recognize that your reason for existence is to pursue the things that excite you the most. The best thing you can do—for yourself and everyone else—is to act on the things you're most passionate about. When you do, you'll shine, and everyone else will see that brilliance.

On a biological level, the mirror neurons of the people around you will activate. They will recognize that they can also follow their dreams and accomplish things they have always wanted to accomplish. On a spiritual level, their souls will remember their reason for being.

I hope you see that you are infinitely capable. You are the entire universe currently perceiving yourself through the eyes of one human. Let's work together to create the world we've always wanted.

Now, with SunMoon Energy, I am working to re-write the narrative of our Earth and the environment. We plan to evolve our species past destructive non-renewable energy sources in favor of green and economically viable self-sustaining power generation technologies.

I have no plans to drink the Mother of the rainforest anytime soon: the lessons from my inaugural three ceremonies continue to grow and I'm confident that I'm on the right path. The way life continues to unfold fills me with the most profound sense of gratitude and I am so thankful for the time I spent in Peru, for Mother Ayahuasca, the shamans, our group, the universe, the creator, and all things. And, I am so thankful for you.

ABOUT MICHAEL SANDERS

Michael Sanders was born March 17, 1987 and grew up in Strathroy, Ontario, Canada. He graduated from Western University with an Honors Degree in Media, Information and Technoculture, along with a Minor in Creative Writing.

In October 2010, Michael lost his best friend, David Edmondson, to a tragic accident which profoundly affected Michael's outlook. He spent a couple of months backpacking through Southeast Asia before moving to Toronto and starting a career in advertising.

As of mid-2015, Michael is the Vice President of ClearMedia advertising agency, in addition to having recently become a partner and the Vice President of Marketing for clean energy and technology startup SunMoon Energy.

Michael has helped many clients earn success through advertising and is now on a mission to help humanity evolve past destructive non-renewable energy in favor of clean energy.

He has also recently launched www.michaelsanders.co, an online resource designed to help you find your enlightenment.

Michael is a passionate traveler, athlete and mover, who regularly practices strength training, Parkour, acrobatics, dance, gymnastics, hand balancing, squash, hiking, and other sports. He believes physical, mental and spiritual health is foundational to a fulfilling life and practices sound nutrition, regular introspection, and daily meditation. He is an avid Burning Man participant and part of the Burner community that extends across the globe. Michael is committed to fostering human connection and improving the world.